TREATING
TRAUMA
SURVIVORS
WITH PTSD

TREATING TRAUMA SURVIVORS WITH PTSD

Edited by

Rachel Yehuda, Ph.D.

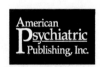

Washington, DC
London, England

Copyright © 2002 American Psychiatric Publishing, Inc.
ALL RIGHTS RESERVED

Manufactured in the United States of America on acid-free paper
10 09 08 07 06   5   4   3   2
First Edition

American Psychiatric Publishing, Inc.
1000 Wilson Boulevard
Arlington, VA 22209-3901
www.appi.org

Library of Congress Cataloging-in-Publication Data
Treating trauma survivors with PTSD / edited by Rachel Yehuda.— 1st ed.
    p. ; cm.
  Includes bibliographical references and index.
  ISBN 1-58562-010-6 (alk. paper)
    1. Post-traumatic stress disorder. I. Yehuda, Rachel.
  [DNLM: 1. Stress Disorders, Post-Traumatic—therapy. 2. Wounds and Injuries—psychology. 3. Survival. WM 170 T7848 2002]
  RC552.P67 T766 2002
  616.85'21—dc21

                                        2001058390

British Library Cataloguing in Publication Data
A CIP record is available from the British Library.

Contents

Contributors

Shawn P. Cahill, Ph.D.
Assistant Professor, Center for the Treatment and Study of Anxiety, University of Pennsylvania School of Medicine, Philadelphia, Pennsylvania

Claude M. Chemtob, Ph.D.
Director, Stress Disorders Laboratory, Pacific Islands Division, National Center for PTSD, Honolulu, Hawaii

Edna B. Foa, Ph.D.
Professor and Director, Center for the Treatment and Study of Anxiety, University of Pennsylvania School of Medicine, Philadelphia, Pennsylvania

Julia Golier, M.D.
Assistant Professor, Traumatic Stress Studies Program, Department of Psychiatry, Mount Sinai School of Medicine, New York, New York

Danny G. Kaloupek, Ph.D.
Associate Professor of Psychiatry and Behavioral Neuroscience, Boston University School of Medicine; Deputy Director, Behavioral Science Division, DVA National Center for PTSD, VA Boston Healthcare System, Boston, Massachusetts

Terence M. Keane, Ph.D.
Professor and Vice Chairman of Research in Psychiatry, Boston University School of Medicine; Director, Behavioral Science Division, DVA National Center for PTSD, VA Boston Healthcare System, Boston, Massachusetts

Alexander C. McFarlane, M.D.
Professor and Head, Department of Psychiatry, University of Adelaide, Adelaide, South Australia

Thomas A. Mellman, M.D.
Associate Professor, Department of Psychiatry, Dartmouth School of Medicine; Director, Psychopharmacology Program, Dartmouth-Hitchcock Medical Center, Lebanon, New Hampshire

Arieh Y. Shalev, M.D.
Professor and Chairman, Department of Psychiatry, Hadassah University Hospital, Jerusalem, Israel

Tisha L. Taylor, Psy.D.
Research Associate, Stress Disorders Laboratory, Pacific Islands Division, National Center for PTSD, Honolulu, Hawaii

Bessel A. van der Kolk, M.D.
Professor of Psychiatry, Boston University School of Medicine; Medical Director, The Trauma Center, Boston, Massachusetts

Rachel Yehuda, Ph.D.
Director, Division of Traumatic Stress, Professor, Department of Psychiatry, Mount Sinai School of Medicine, New York, New York; Director, PTSD Program, VA Medical Center, Bronx, New York

Introduction

Bridging the Gap Between Intervention
Research and Practice

This volume offers a comprehensive examination of issues involved in the treatment of trauma survivors with posttraumatic stress disorder (PTSD). The book summarizes the proceedings of a conference sponsored by the Mount Sinai School of Medicine and held in New York City on September 14, 1999. The program, titled "Advances in the Diagnosis and Treatment of Posttraumatic Stress Disorder," sought to provide a forum for helping clinicians translate the empirical treatment literature into clinical practice through presentations and interactive workshops. This volume tries to capture the dialogue between the treatment literature and clinical practice and, in particular, focus on some of the important issues that are sometimes overlooked in the intervention literature but that are relevant to clinicians who seek to apply treatments described in the literature in real-life clinical settings. Thus, the emphasis is on supplementing and translating the existing intervention literature, rather than directly evaluating specific treatment modalities and their effectiveness. It is our hope that after reading this book, clinicians will have more confidence to apply specialized treatments within the framework of their own practice, regardless of their clinical setting and ideological background.

Most of the contributors have published intervention studies and have formidable clinical experience, making them ideally suited to discuss treatment methods in a way that incorporates an understanding of the complex and often imperfect environment that a clinician must negotiate to deliver services to trauma survivors. Indeed, one issue highlighted in this volume is that the treatment approaches discussed in the empirical literature do not always represent the practices of the clinician. It is sometimes unclear whether this trend represents a call for clinicians to change their practices to match those described in the literature or for researchers to contribute studies to the literature that match treatment techniques that clinicians are using. In the field of PTSD, the majority of intervention studies have examined the efficacy of cognitive-behavioral therapy, particularly exposure therapy. However, only some clinicians routinely use formal exposure therapy in the treatment of PTSD despite its proven efficacy. What are the reasons for this discrepancy between the literature and practice? Do clinicians fail to use specialized treatments because they lack awareness or training in these modalities, or are there realistic considerations that necessitate that other approaches be used? Conversely, does the treatment literature represent a literature of convenience, favoring treatment techniques that are easy to study?

The tension between the literature and clinical practice can be clearly seen in the area of pharmacotherapy. The literature on the pharmacotherapy of PTSD almost exclusively examines the efficacy of single medications against placebo. In practice, however, it is quite common to prescribe two or more medications. In addition, in clinical practice medications are most often used in tandem with psychosocial treatments. However, there are no published studies that have examined the effectiveness of the combined use of psychotherapy and pharmacotherapy. What, then, are the guidelines that direct the clinician in synthesizing knowledge about pharmacotherapy from the literature to a clinical reality that requires usage of multiple medications or a combination of medication with psychotherapy?

Sometimes a treatment becomes widely used before the establishment of an empirical literature that provides evidence for its effectiveness. The applicability of the literature to practice in these cases must also be examined. For example, in the last decade selective serotonin reuptake inhibitors (SSRIs) were used extensively in the clinical treatment of PTSD despite the fact that randomized, double-blind, placebo-controlled studies were (until quite recently) lacking. So too, psychological treatments such as eye movement desensitization reprocessing (EMDR) were widely used by clinicians even before studies began demonstrating the effectiveness of this technique. In both cases, clinical practice strongly guided the intervention literature, which, in turn, provided mixed results on the effectiveness of these treatment approaches. Both SSRIs and EMDR continue to be as commonly used after the emergence of a mixed literature as they were before. This raises the question of the extent to which the empirical findings affect the clinician's behavior, or, conversely, whether clinical practice guides the treatment literature. Regardless, the implications of either possibility in constructing practice guidelines should be examined. These questions highlight the need to examine the relationships among clinical theory, research, and practice.

Another reason that research studies do not always represent clinical practice is that they are performed in environments that differ from those that exist in traditional clinical settings, and possibly in different patients than those who present for clinical treatment. As a result, some of the dilemmas that clinicians face in attempting to treat trauma survivors may not be addressed in treatment studies. Indeed, the exclusion criteria alone for many studies screen out some of the most challenging patients. For example, trauma survivors who are suicidal, who engage in self-destructive behavior, or who are actively abusing substances represent a formidable challenge to clinicians, yet the majority of these trauma survivors would be ineligible for treatment studies until these complicating factors are stabilized. Similarly, in pharmacotherapy studies, the presence of medical illness may also be a reason for excluding the subject from participation. Yet clinicians are often in the position of needing to manage and understand the synergistic effects of mental and physical illnesses in their trauma survivor patients. A question arises then about whether the use of proven treatment techniques is warranted in subjects who have been excluded from participation in research studies.

A related problem concerns the extent to which trauma survivors who are studied in the literature are representative of those who seek treatment in nonresearch settings. In the field of PTSD, the treatments that are being examined are not "experimental" in that they are available to clients who request such treatments and can pay for them. There is often little incentive for a treatment seeker to participate in a research study in which there is either a delay in treatment or the possibility of being randomized into an inert (control) study condition. Furthermore, at least some patients have clear preferences about the kind of modalities that would or would not be acceptable to them. Thus, those who agree to study parameters may be particularly altruistic or intellectually curious, or may have more limited resource options than those who pay for treatment. All these factors may affect the generalizability of the findings.

The need to properly control the experimental environment when doing research is universally appreciated in professional circles, and the more limited inclusion/exclusion criteria in intervention studies are not grounds for invalidating the conclusions of treatment studies. However, an understanding of some of the similarities and differences between subjects recruited for clinical trials and those presenting for treatment is a necessary step in the interpretation of research findings. The awareness that research and clinical environments may be different mandates more guidance in the application of treatments to clinical settings and in addressing whether and how specialized PTSD treatments can be used in the management of patients with more complicated clinical presentations. In addition, there is a need to examine how the clinician should utilize other social and community resources to achieve a more integrated treatment.

Another issue in the translation of the clinical literature to practice is the articulation of the process of how the clinician can come to identify traumatic experiences in their patients and determine the need for specialized trauma-focused treatments. Certainly for mental health providers who specialize in the treatment of trauma survivors (and these are usually among those at the forefront of intervention research), this may be a less salient consideration than for other providers who serve a more general population. For the latter, however, a major obstacle to using specialized treatments is that patients may not present with an awareness that traumatic experiences have occurred in their lives or are relevant to their clinical state. They present with symptoms and problems with coping in their current lives. Often the therapist learns, either in the initial evaluation or during the course of psychotherapy, that the patient has experienced trauma, even though this experience is not formally linked to the reason the patient sought treatment. The difficulty that arises in these cases concerns the negotiation between therapist and patient regarding shifting the focus of the treatment (if it is indicated) to trauma-related issues. Specifically, without a clear mandate from the patient that the therapy be based on examining the impact of a traumatic event, it is difficult to know whether and when specialized trauma-focused treatment techniques should be offered.

In other cases, the patient wants to participate in trauma-focused treatment but presents with a complex symptom pattern that includes PTSD but also symptoms of other conditions. Symptoms related to substance dependence or psychosis may require immediate management and may preclude an exploration of the trauma-related work. However, the empirical intervention literature does not present guidelines about the point at which trauma-related symptoms should be addressed in therapy in patients with multiple problems. The empirical literature also does not address the issue of whether disability claims or pending litigation affect treatment efficacy. Thus, clinicians are often faced with the prospect of deciding whether to use specialized PTSD treatments in these circumstances, to use more traditional methods that might examine the underlying dynamics related to secondary gain, or simply to defer treatment until such matters are resolved.

The decision to use specialized trauma treatment methods may also be complicated in trauma survivors who present after current life stressors. Sometimes the connection between current and past events seems quite clear to the clinician. For example, it is certainly common for a patient to initiate treatment after the death of a spouse or other family member. A clinician may wish to explore whether there is a connection between a current loss and a past trauma, as is often the case, for example, in elderly Holocaust survivors or war veterans. However, it is unclear whether (or when) to deal with the immediate bereavement alone or to frame the symptoms in the larger context of a previous major traumatic event. Although there is considerable anecdotal wisdom regarding how to address all these issues, it is not based on empirical findings.

Despite these unresolved treatment issues, the field of trauma has made considerable advances in the area of assisting clinicians in highlighting proven treatment modalities for those for whom specialized PTSD treatment is clearly warranted. During the past few years, two treatment guidelines have been published: the Expert Consensus Guidelines (Expert Consensus Panels for PTSD 1999) and the treatment guidelines of the International Society for Traumatic Stress Studies (Foa et al. 2000). In the aggregate, these guidelines present an interesting synthesis between expert consensus (Expert Consensus Panels 1999) and findings generated on the basis of empirical evidence (Foa et al. 2000). Indeed, it is suggested that this volume be used as a supplement to these two treatment guidelines.

Treatment guidelines can be helpful in articulating the various treatment modalities available to clinicians, the strength of the evidence for the efficacy of the treatments, and the personal preferences of experts. But, as is more clearly described in Chapter 1, these modalities may require quite a bit of preparatory work by the therapist and patient before beginning these treatments. It is essential to provide information to the clinician to help prepare the patient for trauma-focused work. Specifically, it is imperative to articulate the steps required in helping patients link the trauma with their current symptoms and in helping survivors understand that how they feel now may be related to things that have happened to them in the past. If nothing else, it is essential to point out that such insights are a prerequisite for the use of specialized PTSD treatments and can require a prolonged clinical interaction. Indeed, whereas most clinical trials in the literature last several weeks or months, most clinicians see patients for a more extended period of time, averaging several months or even years. There is a need to resolve the discrepancy between the number of sessions that are stipulated as sufficient for successful PTSD treatment in the literature and the clinical reality that demonstrates a need for extended treatment. This discrepancy can be partially resolved by understanding that the work of engagement and preparation for trauma-focused treatment takes time. Perhaps PTSD treatments should not be considered to have begun until both the therapist and the patient go through a process similar to the informed consent process in which the patient is thoroughly advised of why he or she is eligible for specialized treatments. For realities owing to managed care, it is critical to clarify that this process of engagement is distinct from that of the specialized treatment.

In Chapter 1, Dr. McFarlane and colleagues try to grapple with issues that arise in the treatment planning of trauma survivors that influence, and sometimes mitigate against, the use of specialized PTSD treatment modalities. We discuss a variety of different types of clinical presentations related to trauma exposure and PTSD, including those related to patients with exposure to lower-intensity stressors who present with PTSD symptoms. We also discuss the implications of various comorbid symptoms and disorders in the treatment planning of trauma survivors.

In Chapter 2, Drs. Keane and Kaloupek describe the key components in the diagnosis and assessment of trauma survivors with PTSD and suggest various ways of incorporating research diagnostic instruments into clinical practice for the purpose of evaluation, treatment planning, and monitoring outcomes. Although clinicians may opt to adapt these instruments to fit their own needs, a knowledge of the tools available and familiarity with how to use these instruments can lead to substantial clarification of clinical treatment goals and an operational strategy for knowing when those goals have been met.

Once the diagnosis of PTSD is established, there is a wide array of specialized treatment techniques with proven efficacy that are available tools for the clinician. Treatment guidelines stop short of providing advice about which treatment modalities should be preferentially used. In Chapter 3, Drs. Foa and Cahill tackle the issue of treatment matching. The authors provide a cogent summary of some of the underlying hypotheses and rationales for various treatments and also provide clear explanations of the various treatment approaches that have been highlighted in recent years. They then describe how treatment outcome findings can be used to develop profiles for predicting who is most likely to show remission of symptoms. In Chapter 4, Dr. Mellman provides a comprehensive review of various medications that have been useful in the treatment of PTSD as well as the strength of the empirical evidence for their efficacy. He also discusses some of the inherent biases in how research studies are conducted and evaluated and how these affect translation from the literature to the clinic.

In Chapter 5, Drs. Chemtob and Taylor provide a comprehensive summary of the empirical and clinical literature on the consequences of trauma in children and the efficacy of various treatments. The chapter is particularly helpful in providing a microanalysis of the results of treatment studies, underscoring the strengths and limitations of each study. The authors also discuss differences between the treatment of trauma and its consequences in children and in adults. Finally, the authors provide a conceptual and practical framework to guide single-event child trauma treatment, emphasizing the role of the therapist, clinic, and school environment. This section in particular provides a realistic vision of how therapists can utilize existing community resources to bolster their own clinical interventions.

In Chapter 6, Dr. van der Kolk tackles the problem of assessing and treating complex PTSD. He directly addresses the issue of how the symptoms and treatments of multiply traumatized patients may be different from those of PTSD that results from single or less complex trauma. Dr. van der Kolk makes a compelling case for the fact that although the diverse and complex symptoms in such patients are related to trauma exposure— particularly repeated child abuse—the conventional treatment approaches used in the treatment of PTSD may not provide sufficient relief. This conclusion is based on an explanation of how the biological consequences and developmental disruptions resulting from early trauma are different than those that are present after single-episode stressors in adulthood. Dr. van der Kolk offers important suggestions for the treatment of such individuals that uses approaches that extend beyond those that have been described for the treatment of PTSD.

Finally, in Chapter 7, Dr. Shalev discusses the treatment of trauma survivors in the immediate aftermath of traumatic events. Numerous questions have arisen not only regarding the best treatment modalities for the acute treatment of survivors but also in regard to whether such survivors should be treated at all. At no time in our history have these questions been more relevant to us than in the wake of the September 11 tragedies that have shaken our country. Dr. Shalev advises resolving this dichotomy by reframing the issue in terms of "depth of treatment" and examines the many different needs that acutely traumatized persons have—some of which may require nonpsychological interventions. Although the chapter summarizes existing literature in the treatment of acute trauma, it is clear that this literature is quite limited, yet the need for solutions is great. The chapter also reviews some of the exciting developments in the field regarding the examination of risk factors that influence which trauma survivors are more likely to develop PTSD and therefore are more likely to require treatment in the immediate aftermath of trauma. Normal versus pathological coping response patterns are also described. These descriptions inform clinicians of the prognoses associated with specific behavior and symptom patterns.

Acknowledgments

The conference on which this volume is based arose in response to requests from colleagues in the Division of Traumatic Stress Studies at the Mount Sinai School of Medicine and Bronx Veterans Affairs for more education in applying specialized PTSD treatments. I am grateful to the contributors of this volume, who agreed to teach at the conference in New York and then transcribe their presentations and workshops into written chapters. I am grateful to Pfizer, Inc. for their provision of an unrestricted educational grant for the conference, allowing the program to be offered free of charge to a wide range of local clinicians, and to Innovative Medical Education for their superb work in organizing the conference and preparatory audiotapes for this volume.

I thank Gila Schwarzbaum, M.B.A., for her editorial assistance and Susie Forzano for administrative assistance in the preparation of this volume.

References

Expert Consensus Panels for PTSD: The Expert Consensus Guideline Series. Treatment of posttraumatic stress disorder. J Clin Psychiatry 60(suppl 16):3–76, 1999

Foa EB, Keane T, Friedman MJ: Effective Treatments for PTSD: Practice Guidelines From the International Society for Traumatic Stress Studies. New York, Guilford Press, 2000

1

Treatment Planning for Trauma Survivors With PTSD

What Does a Clinician Need to Know Before Implementing PTSD Treatments?

Alexander C. McFarlane, M.D.
Julia Golier, M.D.
Rachel Yehuda, Ph.D.

Treatment outcome studies provide information about the effectiveness of specific treatments. In practice, however, when formulating a comprehensive treatment plan, clinicians consider many factors above and beyond those related to the empirical data regarding effectiveness in posttraumatic stress disorder (PTSD). This is justified because in clinical practice, trauma survivors may have problems that include but are not limited to PTSD. Furthermore, the goals of the clinician and the patient may differ from those of the researcher. Treatment studies are generally focused on a limited number of outcome measures related to relieving the core symptoms

We thank Drs. Linda Bierer and Ilyse Spertus for their helpful suggestions and editing.

of PTSD. In clinical practice, there may be a whole series of treatment goals—such as improving interpersonal relationships and quality of life and resolving existential issues regarding vulnerability and resilience—that require a broader array of treatments than those described in classic treatment studies.

In addition to possibly having more modest goals, treatment studies operate in a rather circumscribed clinical environment. Most treatment studies are performed within an academic environment and usually do not require the patient to pay for therapy. In clinical practice, however, the treatment plan can be greatly affected by whether and how patients will pay for services. Clinicians operating in health care services such as a Veterans Administration hospital may be able to provide treatment over a long period of time, whereas those operating under the strict aegis of managed care may need to make some very hard decisions regarding which of many clinical problems can be tackled. Practitioners that require self-payment may be faced with other considerations, such as a pressure to produce immediate symptom improvement, even if the improvement is only transient. All clinicians struggle with issues related to the commitment and expectations of patients. In contrast, patients completing clinical trials have shown the requisite commitment to therapy by completing the clinical trial.

Treatment outcome studies are predicated on selecting patients at random, rather than on specific attributes or personal preferences of the treatment seeker. However, the art of clinical practice is to formulate an individualized treatment plan based on unique characteristics of the patient. Thus, the complex step-by-step process of engaging the patient, forming a therapeutic alliance, and negotiating a treatment plan is not operationally addressed in intervention studies. The parallel processes of recruiting, obtaining informed consent, screening, and assessing patients to ascertain study eligibility are not discussed in enough detail in treatment studies to be applicable to clinical practice. In fact, rather than studying the initiation of the treatment relationship, clinical trials begin at the end of this process. The nature of the patient-therapist relationship, and the way in which this is negotiated, can be a critical determinant in creating acceptance of treatment and in predisposing to a successful outcome. Furthermore, because of the pressures of managed care and other regulatory challenges, it has become imperative to articulate this process of engagement and negotiation with the patient to provide insurance companies with more realistic timetables for therapy.

Other barriers to relying too heavily on the treatment literature for treatment planning include the implicit assumptions about the homogeneity of subjects based on the unifying diagnosis of PTSD. The central inclusion criteria for PTSD treatment in clinical trials is the presence of the diagnosis itself. In clinical practice it is the nature of the traumatic event and specific clinical complaint that leads clinicians to choose among the possible interventions and order their introduction. For example, the prominence of intrusive memories may compel a clinician to use cognitive-behavioral therapy, whereas incapacitating depression may require supportive psychotherapy with pharmacologic management. In both cases, diagnostic criteria may be met.

For these reasons, it is essential to bridge the intervention literature and clinical practice with information about the conceptual and practical issues that are involved in therapeutic engagement and treatment planning. The intention of this chapter is to delineate the clinical factors that are not usually described in clinical studies because they involve determinations that are made before having the patient begin the treatment. These variables, however, may greatly influence both whether PTSD treatments are offered and the therapeutic outcome of such treatments. As such, delineating these variables may be helpful in selecting, staging, and supplementing empirically validated treatment modalities. In particular, we focus on issues that are helpful in evaluating the salience of a traumatic event and its relationship to an individual's clinical picture, and on the clinical characteristics at the time of the evaluation that dictate particular clinical directions.

Evaluating the Relationship Between Symptoms and Trauma

To evaluate the extent to which an individual's clinical presentation is a result of exposure to a trauma, it is necessary to know about the event that was experienced. However, many clinicians wonder whether it is appropriate to inquire about traumatic events in the initial meeting with a patient, and if so, how questions about trauma exposure should be asked. Given the statistics that show the enormous prevalence of trauma in our society and in those seeking mental health treatment, it is certainly likely that someone who presents for clinical treatment will have experienced at least one event of sufficient magnitude to quality him or her for a diagnosis of PTSD. Generally, an initial clinical evaluation begins by allowing the patient to present his or her chief complaint. Usually the patient will describe either a series of symptoms or general difficulties in social, occupational, or interpersonal functioning. The time to ask about the presence of either recent or past traumatic events is usually after hearing the patient's description of the current problems. It is natural at this stage to inquire about whether the patient experienced a change in symptoms or functioning after experiencing a major life change or stressor, particularly if the symptoms being identified are among the core symptoms of PTSD. Such inquiry allows the clinician and the patient to consider the extent to which the current symptoms are connected to a recent or past traumatic event. If this is the first meeting, it may not be advisable to ask the patient to expand on the details of the traumatic event, but rather to suggest that part of the work that could be done together might involve an exploration of the impact of the event.

Taking a trauma history early in the evaluation is important because it will help orient both the therapist and the patient to trauma-related issues. It will also demonstrate to the patient that the clinician understands that mental distress may be related to real life events. In fact, the explanation for symptoms offered by the paradigm of trauma often feels reassuring to a person who is sure that his or her problems are self-generated and are due to a constitutional flaw in character, a fundamental weakness, or an inability to cope.

Many trauma survivors present with concerns that they do not recognize as being associated with traumatic stress responses, such as family and vocational problems, and this makes linking symptoms with events even more difficult. Once it is clear that a traumatic event has been sustained, the possibility that current symptoms are related to past events can be entertained. Many trauma survivors present for problems that they do not believe are related to a traumatic event, such as substance abuse or a pre-existing or posttraumatic mood or personality disorder. The clinician must determine not only whether these problems are related to trauma exposure but also whether the solutions to these problems can be found by utilizing specialized PTSD treatments.

Why Trauma Survivors Seek Treatment

For many trauma survivors, reduction of PTSD symptoms may not be the reason for the clinical presentation or even the desired goal of treatment. This is a major consideration in treatment planning. Some trauma survivors may have a comorbid primary psychiatric disorder that is exacerbated by exposure to single or multiple traumatic events. Conditions such as bipolar disorder or psychosis can be exacerbated by trauma. However, in these cases, PTSD treatment may not be warranted, depending on the nature and severity of the other presenting symptoms and the patient's willingness or ability to engage in exploration of trauma-related material.

Some individuals who have been exposed to a major traumatic event in the past may present for treatment after a minor life stress without acknowledging the role that past trauma may have had on current difficulties. A common example is a combat veteran who presents with a grief reaction after a son enlists in the army. In this case, specialized trauma-focused therapy should probably not be undertaken unless it is the expressed wish of the patient to do so. Many trauma survivors seek treatment to alleviate more superficial problems that they believe can in fact be treated, but do not wish to engage in what they perceive to be a more comprehensive ordeal of dredging up the past. Clinicians should build a therapeutic alliance by focusing on a mutually agreed-on set of treatment goals so that the patient will have the opportunity to feel secure in the relationship and the therapeutic process. The clinician should respect the patient's desire to steer away from traumatic material and should frame this as a decision to defer, rather than to avoid, trauma-focused treatment. It is likely that mastery of current issues will enhance the readiness of the patient to engage in therapeutic work that involves the processing of traumatic memories.

Some trauma survivors seek treatment for PTSD even though they do not specifically wish to rid themselves of their PTSD symptoms. Rather, they initially present for treatment to validate their status as trauma survivors. These survivors may be initially resistant to trauma-focused approaches, but rather may first require a series of interventions to examine the meaning of posttraumatic symptoms in their lives. Related to this, some individuals may seek treatment because it is a requirement for obtaining compensation and may actually be threatened by or resistant to treatment that might restore their occupational functioning before settling their claims. It is important for the clinician to help patients articulate why they have come to treatment and what their expectations are from the therapeutic process. The clinician may certainly wish to provide the required evaluation for patients who wish to obtain compensation, and once patients feel secure that these important issues have been addressed, they may be more amenable to examining their resistance to treatment.

Evaluating the Nature of the Trauma

The field of PTSD treatment has emphasized the commonalities inherent in the experience of any trauma rather than the consequences of a particular type of trauma. Such an emphasis has aided in the establishment and the acceptance of the diagnosis of PTSD and has allowed for the development of an integrated subfield within mental health. However, different events may certainly be associated with different types of symptoms and consequences. Empirical research has focused on the relationship between trauma severity and chronicity and the development of PTSD. Stressors that are more severe and chronic are associated with a more complex symptom picture than stressors that are less severe or transitory. Furthermore, stressors involving interpersonal violence (e.g., torture) are thought to involve a far more complex symptom picture than that described within the diagnostic criteria of PTSD (see Chapter 6, this volume). In considering treatment planning, however, survivors may have very different needs depending on what has actually happened in their lives. A person who has recently experienced a natural disaster may require assistance with concrete needs. Psychological interventions may need to focus on issues of loss. In contrast, the trauma of rape may impair intimacy in an already existing relationship and may require interventions that help the survivor deal with issues related to interpersonal trust.

Another factor is whether the individual experienced the trauma alone or with others. Issues of isolation and abandonment may predominate in trauma survivors who experience an event alone. These issues may be quite different than for individuals who have been involved in a traumatic event as part of a group, such as an airplane crash or war. For the latter, feelings related to survivor guilt may be salient, particularly if others experienced a worse fate (or death) at the same time. These considerations may be important in considering individual versus group treatment approaches or in staging of cognitive-behavioral modalities.

Time Elapsed Since the Traumatic Event

When a traumatized person presents to the clinician, it is relevant to inquire about the period of time that has elapsed since the traumatic experience. Although this may not determine the treatment modality that is ultimately chosen, the time elapsed since trauma provides a major window into both diagnosis of the full spectrum of clinical problems and prognosis. The sooner a person presents for treatment after trauma, the clearer the picture of premorbid functioning. The better the premorbid functioning, the more available the person may be for establishing a therapeutic alliance, and the better the outcome of treatment. Poor premorbid functioning may also be related to early trauma exposure. A person traumatized early in life may lack the behavioral repertoire to manage stressful experiences and may require more initial engagement and planning for responses such as dissociation. Importantly, however, recent research is establishing the centrality of pretrauma risk factors in the development of PTSD after trauma. It is often imagined that trauma survivors have led a life free of psychiatric illness and problems before experiencing the focal trauma. However, patients who become disorganized and decompensated after trauma are often those with premorbid psychiatric disturbances and/or previous traumatizations.

In fact, it is important to dispel the notion that if the person presents in the immediate aftermath of a trauma, he or she will have less complex clinical syndromes and less comorbidity. This may not be the case at all. Most trauma survivors who experience symptoms in the immediate aftermath of trauma attempt to live with their suffering for a considerable time before realizing that they will not get better and that there is little choice but to ask for help. People who seek treatment immediately may particularly require support or symptom management as a result of an exacerbation of an existing psychiatric disorder, such as depression. Thus, in treatment planning, attention must be given to preexisting conditions or psychopathology. The idea that survivors simply require acute debriefing or are symptomatic exclusively as a result of a recent event may be naïve.

This is not to say that all survivors who present in the immediate aftermath of trauma have had prior illness. With the increasing awareness of trauma and its consequences, both consumers and clinicians may more carefully monitor the psychological consequences of events and provide education about their short-term and long-term impact. The principles that guide the clinician about the type of interventions required in the immediate aftermath of trauma, and the patients most likely to need these services, are further described in Chapter 7 (this volume). These treatment approaches have in common the goal of preventing symptoms in the immediate aftermath from becoming entrenched and chronic. If the person's distress is settling rapidly, little has to be done other than to monitor the progress of symptom diminution and provide psychoeducation and support. Medications and crisis intervention should also be considered to relieve distress and possibly help with the affective and cognitive distortions that begin to emerge in association with the traumatic memories. The role of benzodiazepines appears to be minimal (Chapter 7, this volume), even though it seems that these agents are often used by clinicians who are responding to patients' manifest distress.

In patients who present for the treatment of PTSD after a trauma that occurred long ago, it is particularly important to determine the immediate circumstances for seeking treatment and to carefully consider the clinical complaint in light of that information. It may be that under the circumstances it is more appropriate to address an issue in the "here and now" rather than embark on an exploration of the past.

Risk Factors

One of the goals of the initial assessment is to determine the role of the traumatic event in producing symptoms. The fact that the majority of individuals do not develop chronic PTSD after a traumatic event suggests that there are risk factors other than exposure to trauma that might be relevant in determining the development of PTSD. This reality compels the clinician to explore issues of vulnerability and other individual characteristics that might be related to why this trauma survivor is symptomatic.

Risk factors for PTSD may include prior traumatization, particularly in childhood; past or contemporaneous psychopathology; psychopathology, particularly PTSD, in the parent of the survivor; cognitive and neurologic abnormalities; and personality traits such as harm avoidance. In considering the presence of these risk factors, the clinician should also entertain the possibility that some risk factors for PTSD may require their own therapeutic interventions.

"Subthreshold" Trauma

DSM-IV (American Psychiatric Association 1994) provides guidelines to help clinicians determine whether an event is severe enough—both objectively and in terms of eliciting a subjective emotional response—to precipitate PTSD. The type of events that are thought to give rise to PTSD are generally those that are directly life-threatening or have the potential to cause death or physical injury. These include, but are not limited to, sexual and physical assault, torture, natural disaster, accidents, and combat. PTSD can develop in persons who experience, witness, or even learn about such events and who react with intense fear, helplessness, or horror at the time of the event.

For reasons that are not entirely clear—but may be related to the link between PTSD and compensation in the legal and forensic arena—many mental health professionals and laypersons are very focused on the objective characteristics of the traumatic events. In determining the presence of PTSD, they can become overly concerned with whether the identified trauma falls within the specified definition articulated in DSM-IV, as if the clinical syndrome of PTSD were based solely on the presence or absence of such an event.

It is indeed common that a patient identifies a stressor in a clinical evaluation that does not meet the criteria for a traumatic stressor because it is not directly or potentially life-threatening. Yet the patient presents with clinical symptoms that are consistent with a diagnosis of PTSD. These cases are usually clinically enigmatic because the prima facie explanation for this presentation is that the patient's reaction appears to be greater than would be expected in response to the particular environmental event. Of course, these cases are less enigmatic for the clinician who is willing to view the DSM-IV as a set of guidelines rather than a bible.

Some illustrative examples of patients presenting with subthreshold events include situations in which the identified event may seem particularly stressful because it is a reminder of a previous traumatic event. For example, Nazi Holocaust survivors may present for treatment in response to issues associated with aging, such as hospitalization due to loss of function. However, under the specter of the Holocaust, these normative processes are tainted with reminders of the fate of others who were too frail to look after themselves. Combat veterans may seem to decompensate when their sons reach the age that they can enter the military, or if their sons make the choice to enter the military. If an individual's response to an environmental stressor seems to be greater than normally expected, the clinician may wish to explore earlier events that may be the true source of the distress being experienced, of which the current stressor may be a reminder.

In some cases it is difficult to ascertain whether there is a prior trauma or whether the patient is simply showing an exaggerated response to a stressor that most individuals would not find traumatic. The clinician should never insist that a prior trauma must be present to justify such an exaggerated emotional response to an event. In fact, because it is now recognized that a variety of vulnerability factors are associated with the development of PTSD, the presence of risk factors could certainly explain why some people develop symptoms to lower-magnitude events. Although there is generally a relationship between the severity of PTSD and that of the traumatic event, PTSD can also develop in response to less traumatic events. This implies that vulnerability factors may be particularly important farther down the spectrum of horror and catastrophe. If lower-magnitude traumatic events are more likely to lead to PTSD under conditions of increased vulnerability, then vulnerable individuals might show exaggerated responses to "subthreshold" stressful events.

If the clinician believes that a PTSD syndrome is present even if the traumatic event is subthreshold, then he or she should embark on a treatment plan that uses specialized PTSD treatments and should attempt to address vulnerability factors even if the criteria of PTSD are not met.

Behavior of the Patient During the Interview

The treatment that is ultimately implemented is optimally determined by the patient's mental state and his or her capacity to manage the interview process, particularly as it relates to trauma-based associations. The initial assessment process gives the clinician an opportunity to gauge how the patient will tolerate exposure to trauma-related material.

Trauma-Related Distress

In the process of taking an initial history, the clinician has an opportunity to observe the potential disruption of a person's demeanor or equanimity simply by monitoring his or her reaction to talking about traumatic experiences. The clinician quickly becomes aware of the patient's ability to contain and/or modulate the distress associated with a traumatic memory. There are some patients who are able to give little of the history of a traumatic event before becoming overwhelmed by the reemergence of feelings of horror or helplessness. On the other hand, others show withdrawal and avoidance, which may equally signal intolerable distress. On further questioning a clinician might learn that this withdrawal is a response to the arousal of intense affective states associated with the recollection of components of the traumatic experience. In contrast, such withdrawal might also imply a dissociative state or a more generalized depression. Evidence of intense arousal or negative mood is an indication that pharmacologic intervention may be warranted. Medication in this early phase of treatment planning may help stabilize a patient to enable him or her to learn behavioral strategies to modulate anxiety and PTSD symptoms. For patients who do not like the idea of taking a medication at an early stage of treatment, psychoeducation should be used to help the patient understand the symptoms of PTSD in the context of a biological response to stress. Because medication of PTSD will likely require months rather than weeks, it is particularly necessary to engage in a mutual decision about pharmacotherapy for a patient who is reluctant about this modality.

Dissociation

The process of focusing on trauma-related memories can cause some patients to undergo varying degrees of dissociation. This may happen before or after the interview, when the clinician is not present and cannot act as an aid to orientation. Suspicion about dissociation may be triggered by the patient arriving late for appointments because of uncharacteristically getting lost, or by the patient displaying a general sense of disorganization. Dissociative responses may follow a particular trigger of the traumatic memory or can be precipitated by questions about historical facts. Patients who seem confused about specific aspects of events that have occurred or who state that they have forgotten large chunks of salient autobiographical information may similarly be experiencing dissociation. When treating such patients, clinicians are often concerned that a direct engagement regarding the trauma will intensify the dissociation. As a result, clinicians sometimes move away from traumatic material more than is clinically necessary because they respond to the patient's fear of being unable to reconstitute after such a response.

The strategies for initiating therapy with dissociative patients are similar to those employed for patients who are highly distressed. It is sometimes useful to conceptualize dissociation as arising from unmodulated anxiety and as a secondary, reactive process evoked in the service of maintaining a state of emotional homeostasis. Thus, strategies that help the patient anticipate increased arousal and manage its emergence are important first steps in the treatment, as are strategies that focus on helping the patient stay in the here and now. In other words, a patient who is beginning to dissociate during the recall of a traumatic memory can be taught to identify his or her surroundings and to shift focus from the past to the current reality. Medication is also useful in modulating the patient's anxiety and diminishing the propensity to dissociate. These interventions often make trauma-related material more accessible while reducing its disorganizing potential.

Emotional Numbing and Withdrawal

Engagement with both the therapist and the traumatic memory is a necessary requirement to initiate change. However, many patients present for treatment in a state of emotional withdrawal and detachment, and some are frankly alexithymic. Even with direct clinical probing, very little of their trauma history or associated mental states can be readily ascertained. Although patients may report times when the traumatic memory intrudes and causes distress, such as in nightmares, they may do so in a flat monotone, thereby masking their internal distress and anxiety, and resulting in the clinician minimizing their problems.

Furthermore, for a patient who presents as unemotional, the chief complaint may be in the nature of an existential dilemma regarding the trauma, which may be a consequence of this state of detachment and noninvolvement. Such patients may frequently intellectualize about inhumanity or distant atrocities perpetrated around the world, but even these complaints are made in a nonemotional way and convey resignation and a lack of hope. Relationships with family and friends are described as superficial and largely devoid of intimacy. It is difficult for such patients to articulate the extent to which this numbness is actively distressing for them, and instead they talk about seemingly irrelevant material. Their inability to verbalize their distress is sometimes interpreted by the clinician as an unwillingness to engage in trauma-related work. The challenge of working with such patients is to engage and maintain them in a therapeutic relationship with the goal of making their inner psychological states more accessible to reflection. These patients are quite a bit more challenging than those who present with intense distress, but this is only because it is often difficult to see the intense distress or to engage the patient in discussions about it. Detachment is a mental state that is a predictor of poor outcome in conventional exposure-based treatments (see Chapter 3, this volume). Getting to the point where reflection is possible requires a two-step process in which the first step involves addressing the immediate relationships of the individual to highlight issues that lead to interpersonal conflict. Although it may certainly be the case that the issues that promote such conflict also elicit traumatic memories, the patient can be more readily engaged by first examining ways in which he or she can strengthen interpersonal ties. This has the added benefit of shoring up the patient's ability to use interpersonal relationships as support systems. The patient can subsequently be guided to examine how conflict more generally promotes internal trauma-related distress, which is the second stage of the process.

Thus, the process of engagement requires the therapist to help the patient notice that conflicts that arise within important immediate relationships are actually mini-triggers for trauma-related material and that the ensuing interpersonal withdrawal is a type of trauma avoidance. Development of a trusting relationship with the therapist is central to the treatment of someone with emotional numbing. Sharing feelings, even with the therapist, becomes a vehicle for allowing the patient to recognize that his or her ability to have intimate feelings is still intact, despite the emotional distancing from loved ones. Similarly, group therapy can provide a further opportunity for trauma survivors to learn to express feelings toward each other. The difference between such engagements and classic psychodynamic therapy that relies on transference interpretations and analysis of interpersonal dynamics is that in the context of trauma-focused work this type of engagement is being used as a vehicle to access traumatic material and not as an end in itself.

Interpersonal Vigilance

Some traumatic experiences involve direct interpersonal violence, injury, or death. This type of trauma often leaves the survivor in a state in which almost any relationship, including that with the therapist, becomes a potential traumatic reminder. In these patients, a prolonged engagement may be contraindicated and may only serve to further distance the patient from therapy. Rather, giving patients concrete behavioral tools to empower them may provide them with a sense of a greater sense of security and control. In fact, there are cases in which classic psychodynamic approaches only serve to entrench a patient in maladaptive defensive patterns, particularly because they may maintain avoidance. In cases where the traumatic image is clearly expressed as troublesome, the early introduction of exposure therapy can be useful. This also helps in restoring accurate perceptions of the world. Ultimately, these interventions establish safety, which is a requirement for symptom resolution.

Explosive Anger

Some patients present requesting assistance in managing specific behaviors associated with PTSD such as irritability and feelings of uncontrollable anger. In these cases, patients should be directed to anger management before beginning traumatic memory work. This approach necessitates the implementation of steps to identify triggers to aggression and the development of strategies to modulate early reactions to conflict. Although patients presenting with aggression are often relieved to hear that this behavior can be trauma related, they should ideally be educated about the necessity of making anger management one of the first priorities of treatment. Successful anger management may or may not require subsequent trauma-focused work. This determination should be made during a reevaluation phase after behavioral control has been attained.

Suicidal Thinking and Risk-Taking Behavior

The association between self-destructive behavior and trauma has received less attention in the research literature than is warranted, given the clinical importance of the problem. One view is that this apparent neglect results from the difficulty of conducting research with erratic and impulsive patients. Because these patients are not generally included in treatment studies, they are not the subject of discussion in the treatment literature. It is also possible that the potential stigma associated with suicidal or self-harming behavior has also prompted trauma survivors and clinicians to view this behavior as comorbid rather than a direct consequence of exposure. The debate over whether disorders of extreme stress not otherwise specified or complex PTSD (van der Kolk et al. 1996) should be included in DSM-IV centered around whether such behavior was a specific aspect of the trauma response or was associated with other (mood or personality) disorders (see Chapter 6, this volume). Regardless, in clinical practice, suicidal ideation and risk-taking behavior can emerge and must be dealt with seriously before any trauma-focused interventions commence.

It is helpful to understand that suicidal and risk-taking or self-harming behavior tends to occur in those who are overwhelmed by negative affect. However, there may not be sufficient time for the therapist to help patients "understand" these behaviors. Initially, the therapist must make a comprehensive evaluation of the suicidal ideation or behavior, particularly with respect to severe depressive illness, which increases the risk of completed suicide. The interpretation of suicidal gestures, on the other hand, is more complex and may indicate longstanding personality or affective instability. In the latter instance, clinicians usually recommend behavioral interventions that are geared toward teaching patients to modulate affect, such as dialectic behavioral therapy or other interventions that have been useful with patients with personality disorder. For more information about treatment approaches for such patients, see Chapter 6 (this volume). For treatment planning, however, the clinician should emphasize the importance of developing and practicing various methods of self monitoring. The identification of safety strategies that can be recruited at times of significant distress is critical to the beginning stages of treatment in patients who present with such difficulties. To address affective instability and risk-taking behavior, pharmacologic interventions should also be considered.

Psychiatric Comorbidity

The issue of psychiatric comorbidity has received little attention in the treatment literature, possibly owing to the restricted admission criteria for entry into most treatment studies. In this regard, there is an interesting dichotomy between the treatment literature and the literature on phenomenology and pathophysiology of PTSD. The treatment literature has generally excluded patients with comorbidity, whereas studies of phenomenology and pathophysiology have emphasized that psychiatric comorbidity is the rule, rather than the exception, in trauma survivors with PTSD (Kessler et al. 1995). Part of the dilemma is that before a treatment—particularly a pharmacologic one—is considered effective for PTSD it must often be demonstrated that its effectiveness is not a secondary consequence of symptom reduction of another disorder such as depression.

The question is whether to treat dually diagnosed individuals with PTSD treatment modalities hoping that the other conditions will improve as a result of such therapy, or whether to formulate a treatment plan that addresses comorbid disorders separately. If the latter option is preferable, the next question that arises concerns the staging of different treatments.

The answers to these questions depend on the nature, severity, and pattern of the comorbid diagnosis. Defining the temporal relationship of the emergence of comorbid disorders to PTSD is of primary importance in determining how they should be addressed in treatment. Certainly, disorders that may have been present before the development of PTSD—or even before trauma exposure—may require interventions independent of those targeting PTSD symptoms.

One of the strategies in addressing comorbidity is to select a treatment that might be clinically indicated for both (or all) the disorders present. In fact, the value of addressing diagnoses simultaneously with selective serotonin reuptake inhibitors has been suggested by Brady et al. (1995), who found that sertraline decreased both PTSD symptoms and alcohol consumption in patients dually diagnosed with PTSD and alcoholism. Similarly, in a study of female patients taking methadone, Hien and Levin (1994) found that not treating patients for comorbid symptoms of PTSD hindered treatment response and tended to be associated with increased dropout rates, emergent depressive symptoms, and new substance abuse. Kofoed and coworkers (1993) concluded that PTSD and substance abuse should be treated simultaneously and that the effectiveness of drug and alcohol treatment is decreased by the existence of extreme psychological symptoms. Thus, appropriate management of comorbid psychiatric symptoms tends to improve the outcome of substance abuse treatment.

In some individuals who have been exposed to extremely traumatic events, the comorbid disorder rather than the PTSD can dominate the clinical picture. The individual can present with severe depressive symptoms with traumatic ruminations being an important but relatively secondary component. This is in contrast to the individual whose intrusive recollections and associated hyperarousal are the immediate symptoms for which the person seeks treatment. Both psychotherapeutic and pharmacologic strategies should be employed with the aim of reducing subjective distress sufficiently to permit trauma-focused work to proceed.

It is unlikely that the symptoms of a comorbid psychiatric condition will improve merely by addressing the PTSD using nonpharmacologic interventions unless the comorbid condition is clearly a secondary consequence of PTSD or unless the same treatment is indicated for both disorders. In a population of adolescents, Goenjian et al. (1997) examined the effect of a brief trauma- and grief-focused psychotherapy program after the 1988 earthquake in Armenia. In follow-up assessments 1.5 and 3 years after the earthquake, the researchers found that psychotherapy had significantly decreased emergent symptoms of posttraumatic stress. Although there had been no change in the severity of the depressive symptoms in subjects treated with trauma-focused psychotherapy, the depressive symptoms among those not treated had significantly worsened with time. This is an interesting population-based study emphasizing that a trauma-focused treatment may not improve depressive symptoms in the short term, and it underscores the necessity of providing primary treatment for both disorders, when indicated.

Core Competencies in the Treatment of PTSD

A central component of delivering effective treatment of PTSD is to have access to a range of clinical skills. In addition, the clinician should have a good working knowledge of relevant treatment modalities even if he or she is not in a position to implement them. That is, the non-M.D. clinician should have a basic understanding of the pharmacotherapy of PTSD and a physician should undergo the different types of psychotherapy, even if he or she does not conduct them. If a clinician finds himself or herself using the same treatment approaches with each PTSD patient, this might ultimately suggest that the clinician is using techniques of convenience (i.e., ones that he or she is familiar with) rather than those that are actually clinically warranted. If a non-M.D. clinician finds that medications are never warranted in PTSD treatment, this would be an occurrence that requires self-reflection. Although it may seem daunting to continually learn new treatment approaches or to seek to extend one's knowledge, it is a clinician's responsibility to be aware of new options and, whenever possible, to learn to apply them to clinical practice. Alternatively, developing a network of colleagues that complement a clinician's skills can be quite helpful. Clinicians working as part of a team with others possessing a range of skills ensures the best outcome for patients. However, even if the clinician does not have mastery over the application of specific techniques, he or she must be able to understand when the use of such techniques is warranted.

Central Aspects of Treatment

Whatever technique is ultimately used, the rationale of therapy with traumatized patients must be communicated as part of the development of a treatment plan. This involves highlighting that the aim is to help them move from being haunted by the past and interpreting subsequent emotionally arousing stimuli as a return of the trauma, to being present in the here and now, capable of responding to current exigencies to their fullest potential. To do that, treatment assists them to regain control over their emotional responses and place the trauma in the larger perspective of their lives—as a historical event, or series of events, that occurred at a particular time and place. The key element of the psychotherapy of people with PTSD is the integration of the alien, the unacceptable, the terrifying, and the incomprehensible. Life events initially experienced as alien, imposed from outside on passive victims, must come to be personalized as integrated aspects of one's history and life experiences (van der Kolk and Ducey 1989). The defenses initially established as emergency protective measures must gradually relax their grip on the psyche, so that dissociated aspects of experience do not continue to intrude into the individual's life experience, thereby threatening to retraumatize an already traumatized person.

Psychotherapy must address two fundamental aspects of PTSD: 1) deconditioning of anxiety and 2) altering the way survivors view themselves and their world by reestablishing a feeling of personal integrity and control. In only the simplest cases will it be sufficient to decondition the anxiety associated with the trauma. In the vast majority of patients, both aspects need to be treated. This means the use of a combination of procedures for deconditioning anxiety, for reestablishing a personal sense of control (which can range from engaging in physical challenges to reestablishing a sense of spiritual meaning), and forming meaningful and mutually satisfying relationships with others (often by means of group psychotherapy).

There is a need to understand more about the process of engaging in treatment and the issues behind the acceptability of various approaches. It may be that traumatic events have a particular capacity to disrupt relationships, and this is a major impediment to engaging in treatment. The issue of the engagement of the patient and dealing with loss is especially important in cases in which there has been a traumatic bereavement. The intervention needs to address the matter of grief as well as the traumatic memories. The clinician's role in providing general information and specific education about symptoms also makes a contribution to the patient's improvement (McFarlane 1994). The best ways to implement this role and the ways that it affects the outcome of cognitive and exposure treatments are also important questions. Particular attention is required if the patient has also sustained a traumatic injury, as discussed above. Often the association between these somatic symptoms and the trauma is not directly expressed by the patient. Careful physical examination can elicit these phenomena and the triggers that intensify the symptoms. In addition, the need to demonstrate improvement does not address the issue of chronic and disabling illness, in which the prevention of decline is a more realistic goal. Hence it is not possible to have a simple algorithm that defines the most appropriate treatment plan with a PTSD patient.

References

American Psychiatric Association: Diagnostic and Statistical Manual of Mental Disorders, 4th Edition. Washington, DC, American Psychiatric Association, 1994

Brady KT, Sonne SC, Roberts JM: Sertraline treatment of comorbid posttraumatic stress disorder and alcohol dependence. J Clin Psychiatry 56(11):502–505, 1995

Goenjian AK, Karayan I, Pynoos RS, et al: Outcome of psychotherapy among early adolescents after trauma. Am J Psychiatry 154(4):536–542, 1997

Hien D, Levin FR: Trauma and trauma-related disorders for women on methadone: prevalence and treatment considerations. J Psychoactive Drugs 26(4): 421–429, 1994

Kessler RC, Bromet E, Hughes M, et al: Posttraumatic stress disorder in the National Comorbidity Survey. Arch Gen Psychiatry 52, 1048–1060, 1995

Kofoed L, Friedman MJ, Peck R: Alcoholism and drug abuse in patients with PTSD. Psychiatr Q 64(2):151–171, 1993

McFarlane AC: Individual psychotherapy of posttraumatic stress disorder. Psychiatr Clin North Am 17(2):393–408, 1994

van der Kolk BA, Ducey CP: The psychological processing of traumatic experience: Rorschach patterns in PTSD. J Trauma Stress 2(3):259–274, 1989

van der Kolk BA, Weisaeth L, van der Hart O: History of trauma in psychiatry, in Traumatic Stress: The Effects of Overwhelming Experience on Mind, Body and Society. Edited by van der Kolk BA, McFarlane AC, Weisaeth L. New York, Guilford Press, 1996, pp 47–74

Additional Reading

American Psychiatric Association: Diagnostic and Statistical Manual of Mental Disorders. Washington, DC, American Psychiatric Association, 1952

American Psychiatric Association: Diagnostic and Statistical Manual of Mental Disorders, 3rd Edition. Washington, DC, American Psychiatric Association, 1980

Australian Bureau of Statistics: Mental Health and Wellbeing: Profile of Adults—Australia, 1997. Canberra, Australia, Australian Bureau of Statistics, 1998

Bion WR: Experiences in Groups. London, Tavistock, 1961

Breuer J, Freud S: Psychical mechanisms of hysterical phenomena: preliminary communication, in Studies on Hysteria, Vol 3. Harmondsworth, England, Penguin Books, 1893

Brom D, Kleber RJ, Hofman MC: Victims of traffic accidents: incidence and prevention of post-traumatic stress disorder. J Clin Psychol 49(2):131–140, 1993

Caplan G: Principles of Preventive Psychiatry. New York, Basic Books, 1964

Davidson JRT: Biological therapies for posttraumatic stress disorder: an overview. J Clin Psychiatry 58(suppl 9):29–32, 1997

Foa EB: Psychological processes related to recovery from trauma and an effective treatment for PTSD. Ann N Y Acad Sci 821:410–424, 1997

Foa EB, Kozak MJ: Emotional processing of fear: exposure to corrective information. Psychol Bull 99(1):20–35, 1986

Foa EB, Rothbaum BO, Riggs DS, Murdock TB: Treatment of posttraumatic stress disorder in rape victims: a comparison between cognitive-behavioural procedures and counselling. J Consult Clin Psychol 59(5):715–725, 1991

Freud S: The Standard Edition of the Complete Psychological Works of Sigmund Freud, Vol 7. Translated and edited by Strachey J. London, Hogarth Press, 1955

Hafferty FW, Light DW: Professional dynamics and the changing nature of medical work. J Health Soc Behav (Spec No):132–153, 1995

Horowitz MJ: Stress Response Syndromes. New York, Jason Aronson, 1976

Janet P: L'Automatisme Psychologique. Paris, Alcan, 1889

Justice B: Alternative medicine's relevance to public health practice and research. Altern Ther Health Med 2(3):24–25, 1996

Kaplan HI, Sadock BJ (eds): Comprehensive Textbook of Psychiatry/VI. Baltimore, MD, Williams & Wilkins, 1995

Keane TM, Kaloupek DG: Imaginal flooding in the treatment of a posttraumatic stress disorder. J Consult Clin Psychol 50(1):138–140, 1982

Keenan B: An Evil Cradling. London, Vintage, 1993

Kulka R, Schlenger WE, Fairbank JA, et al: Trauma and the Vietnam War generation: report of the findings from the National Vietnam Veterans' readjustment study. New York, Brunner/Mazel, 1990

Lindemann E: Symptomatology and management of acute grief. Am J Psychiatry 101:141–148, 1944

McFarlane AC: On the social denial of trauma and the problem of not knowing the past, in International Handbook of Human Response to Trauma. Edited by Shalev A, Yehuda R, McFarlane A. New York, Kluwer Academic/Plenum Publishers, 2000

Rabkin JG, Struening, EL: Life events stress and mental illness. Science 194:1013–1020, 1976

Raphael B: Preventive intervention with the recently bereaved. Arch Gen Psychiatry 34(12):1450–1454, 1977

Raphael B: When Disaster Strikes. New York, Basic Books, 1986

Resick PA, Schnicke NK: Cognitive processing therapy for sexual assault victims. J Consult Clin Psychol 60(5):748–756, 1992

Shapiro F: EMDR: evaluation of controlled PTSD research. J Behav Ther Exp Psychiatry 27(3):209–218, 1996

Singh B, Raphael B: Postdisaster support of the bereaved. A possible role for preventive psychiatry? J Nerv Ment Dis 169(4):203–212, 1981

Sparr LF, Moffitt MC, Ward MF: Missed psychiatric appointments: who returns and who stays away? Am J Psychiatry 150:801–805, 1993

Uhlenhuth EH, Balter MB, Ban TA, et al: International Study of Expert Judgement on Therapeutic Use of Benzodiazepines and Other Therapeutic Medications: V. Treatment strategies in panic disorder, 1992–1997. J Clin Psychopharmacol 18(6 suppl 2):27S–31S, 1998

van der Kolk BA: Foreword, in Countertransference in the Treatment of PTSD. Edited by Wilson JP, Lindy JD. New York, Guilford Press, 1994, pp vii–xii

Weisaeth L: PTSD: vulnerability and protective factors. Bailliere's Clinical Psychiatry 2(2):217–228, 1996

Wilson M: DSM-III and the transformation of American psychiatry: a history. Am J Psychiatry 150:399–410, 1993

2

Diagnosis, Assessment, and Monitoring Outcomes in PTSD

Terence M. Keane, Ph.D.
Danny G. Kaloupek, Ph.D.

Posttraumatic stress disorder (PTSD) was first included in the diagnostic nomenclature of the American Psychiatric Association in 1980. Since that time, there has been excellent progress in the psychological assessment of PTSD. PTSD is a psychological condition that can develop in individuals after exposure to major life stressors (American Psychiatric Association 1994) and is characterized by a range of symptoms. Among the prominent symptoms of PTSD are distressing thoughts, feelings, and images that recapitulate the traumatic event, a persistent avoidance of cues associated with the traumatic event, emotional numbing of responsiveness, and a collection of symptoms that represent a persistent increase in stress and arousal. Typically, the disturbance is experienced for longer than 1 month and causes clinically significant distress or impairment in occupational and social functioning. Capturing the diversity of symptoms in PTSD has constituted a significant challenge to those involved in the development of assessment instruments. Yet it is clear that this challenge has been successfully met with an assortment of diagnostic interviews and psychological tests (Keane et al. 2000).

For a diagnosis of PTSD to be made, an individual must have been exposed to a traumatic event that involved a life-endangering component. The individual's response had to include intense fear, helplessness, or horror. If symptom duration is less than 3 months, acute PTSD is diagnosed; if duration extends beyond 3 months, the condition is considered to be chronic. In some individuals, symptoms emerge months or even years after the traumatic event. In these cases a diagnosis of PTSD with delayed onset is considered.

Diagnostic Criteria for PTSD

Fortunately, most people who are exposed to a traumatic event recover over time. For a sizable minority, however, symptoms of PTSD occur and in the absence of treatment can cascade into the development of a persistent and disabling psychiatric condition. A person with PTSD reexperiences symptoms that include recurrent and intrusive recollections of the event; recurrent dreams of the event; feeling as if the event were recurring; intense distress at exposure to cues that symbolize the event; and physiologic reactivity to cues or reminders of the event (Table 2–1).

The disorder also encompasses symptoms of avoidance and emotional numbing. These can include efforts to avoid thoughts, feelings, or even conversations of the event; efforts to avoid activities, places, or people associated with the event; an inability to recall important details surrounding the event; a diminished interest in formerly enjoyable activities of life; a feeling of detachment, estrangement, or alienation from other people; a restricted range of emotional experiences; and a sense of a shortened future accompanied by a notable lack of preparation for the future.

In addition, symptoms of arousal that were not present before the traumatic event complete the symptom picture. These arousal symptoms can be sleep problems, irritability or anger outbursts, difficulty concentrating, hypervigilance for danger or a recurrence of a life-threatening situation, or exaggerated startle response.

Relevance of Traumatic Events

Although it was formerly thought that exposure to traumatic events was rare, recent epidemiological research has challenged this notion. Norris (1992) studied four urban areas in the southern United States and found that 69% of adults reported experiencing one or more traumatic events in their lives. Resnick et al. (1993) conducted a nationwide survey of victimization among women and found that 69% reported being victimized at least once in their lives. Breslau et al. (1991) found that 39% of participants in their epidemiological study experienced a traumatic event. These participants were a relatively young, well-educated, and insured population. Even college student populations reported high rates of exposure to trau-

TABLE 2-1.	DSM-IV-TR diagnostic criteria for PTSD

A. The person has been exposed to a traumatic event in which both of the following were present:

    (1) the person experienced, witnessed, or was confronted with an event or events that involved actual or threatened death or serious injury, or a threat to the physical integrity of self or others

    (2) the person's response involved intense fear, helplessness, or horror. **Note:** In children, this may be expressed instead by disorganized or agitated behavior.

B. The traumatic event is persistently reexperienced in one (or more) of the following ways:

    (1) recurrent and intrusive distressing recollections of the event, including images, thoughts, or perceptions. **Note:** In young children, repetitive play may occur in which themes or aspects of the trauma are expressed.

    (2) recurrent distressing dreams of the event. **Note:** In children, there may be frightening dreams without recognizable content.

    (3) acting or feeling as if the traumatic event were recurring (includes a sense of reliving the experience, illusions, hallucinations, and dissociative flashback episodes, including those that occur on awakening or when intoxicated). **Note:** In young children, trauma-specific reenactment may occur.

    (4) intense psychological distress at exposure to internal or external cues that symbolize or resemble an aspect of the traumatic event

    (5) physiological reactivity on exposure to internal or external cues that symbolize or resemble an aspect of the traumatic event

C. Persistent avoidance of stimuli associated with the trauma and numbing of general responsiveness (not present before the trauma), as indicated by three (or more) of the following:

    (1) efforts to avoid thoughts, feelings, or conversations associated with the trauma

    (2) efforts to avoid activities, places, or people that arouse recollections of the trauma

    (3) inability to recall an important aspect of the trauma

    (4) markedly diminished interest or participation in significant activities

    (5) feeling of detachment or estrangement from others

    (6) restricted range of affect (e.g., unable to have loving feelings)

    (7) sense of a foreshortened future (e.g., does not expect to have a career, marriage, children, or a normal life span)

D. Persistent symptoms of increased arousal (not present before the trauma), as indicated by two (or more) of the following:

    (1) difficulty falling or staying asleep

    (2) irritability or outbursts of anger

    (3) difficulty concentrating

    (4) hypervigilance

    (5) exaggerated startle response

TABLE 2–1.	DSM-IV-TR diagnostic criteria for PTSD *(continued)*

E. Duration of the disturbance (symptoms in Criteria B, C, and D) is more than 1 month.

F. The disturbance causes clinically significant distress or impairment in social, occupational, or other important areas of functioning.

Specify if:

    Acute: if duration of symptoms is less than 3 months

    Chronic: if duration of symptoms is 3 months or more

Specify if:

    With Delayed Onset: if onset of symptoms is at least 6 months after the stressor

Source. Reprinted from American Psychiatric Association: *Diagnostic and Statistical Manual of Mental Disorders*, 4th Edition, Text Revision. Washington, DC, American Psychiatric Association, 2000. Copyright 2000, American Psychiatric Association. Used with permission.

matic events. Vrana and Lauterbach (1994) found that 84% of the undergraduate population at a major Midwestern university reported exposure, with 33% stating that they had experienced four or more traumatic events. Clearly, exposure to traumatic events is a common event in the lives of adult Americans.

National Prevalence of PTSD

Clearly, people who are exposed to traumatic life events do not always develop PTSD. In the study by Breslau et al. (1991), approximately 25% of those exposed to a traumatic event ultimately developed PTSD, resulting in a lifetime prevalence of nearly 9%. Norris (1992) found a current prevalence rate of PTSD of 5%, whereas Resnick and colleagues (1993) reported a 9% current rate of PTSD among women accompanied by a 12% lifetime rate. General-population estimates have also yielded high rates of PTSD. In Kessler and colleagues' (1995) National Comorbidity Survey, lifetime PTSD was found in 8% of the adult population.

Prevalence rates of PTSD in children have received little empirical attention to date; this is an area in clear need of additional research. Impeding progress in this area is a distinct lack of diagnostic measurement tools that reliably and validly evaluate PTSD in children. Among adolescents, the prevalence of PTSD was measured in a recent study by Kilpatrick and Saunders (1999). Using a nationwide probability sampling strategy, they found that PTSD was as common in adolescents as it is in adults, with estimates reaching 8%. Also similar to the adult population, PTSD in adolescence was more common among girls and minority groups. Moreover, the prevalence of PTSD increased linearly as the number of traumatic events increased. The consistency of this linear relationship of exposure to traumatic events and the development of PTSD across populations, studies, and measurement tools strongly supports the key role that social and contextual factors play in the development of psychological disturbance.

PTSD also seems to occur at higher rates in populations that we characterize as high risk for the disorder. The National Vietnam Veterans Readjustment Study (NVVRS; Kulka et al. 1990), a landmark epidemiological effort that was the first attempt by any country to quantify the psychological toll of a war on its soldiers, found that 30% of the 3.1 million Vietnam veterans developed PTSD at some time after the war. This represented some 958,000 cases of PTSD just from the Vietnam War. Fifteen percent (479,000) of these veterans still had PTSD 15 years after the conclusion of the war.

Similarly, individuals who have experienced rape are also at greater risk for developing PTSD. Kilpatrick and colleagues' (1992) National Women's Study found that 13% of American women had experienced a completed rape at some time in their lives. Nearly a third of them eventually developed PTSD as a result. This study yielded a strikingly high national prevalence rate of 4% for rape-related PTSD among American women.

Disasters also seem to induce PTSD at high rates. Green and colleagues (1992) studied the effects of the dam collapse in Buffalo Creek, West Virginia. They found a 59% lifetime rate of PTSD among survivors and a 25% current rate 14 years after the flooding.

The role of traumatic events and PTSD in the national problem of homelessness has recently been highlighted. The Better Homes Fund (1999) examined the rates of violence in the lives of homeless mothers and children and found staggering rates of physical and sexual abuse. Ninety-two percent of homeless mothers have been severely physically or sexually abused either as adults or as children. This abuse was typically at the hands of an intimate partner or a caregiver. Thirty-six percent of homeless mothers had diagnostic criteria for PTSD—three times the national rate for women in the general population. Although causality cannot be inferred from these correlational data, this study has generated important hypotheses about the possible impact of traumatic experiences and PTSD on the growing problem of homeless families.

Clearly, exposure to traumatic events is common in the United States, and it seems that the prevalence of PTSD in the general population is high, ranking in frequency behind only alcohol abuse, major depression, and social phobia. As a result, trauma exposure and PTSD represent a major challenge to the health care delivery system.

Most research on the prevalence of traumatic events and PTSD has been conducted in the United States. Many scholars believe that the prevalence of trauma exposure and PTSD is higher in the developing world, in part due to the lack of resources present there to avert disasters and to mitigate their aftermath (De Girolamo et al. 1996). Future research will determine the extent to which this is an accurate assessment of the situation in developing countries.

Gender differences in exposure and in the development of PTSD are suggested by the results of several epidemiological studies. It seems that males (60%) are more likely to be exposed to traumatic events than are females (50%), as was found in the National Comorbidity Survey (Kessler et al. 1995). Yet females are more likely to develop PTSD (12%) than are males (6%). This distinction may well be a real gender difference in the susceptibility to PTSD, possibly linked to biological, psychological, or social differences. Alternatively, it may be a direct function of the types of events to which men and women are differentially exposed. For example, women are more than 10 times as likely to be raped and men are twice as likely to have experienced a dangerous accident. The capacity of different events to induce PTSD at different rates is only now being explored systematically. These studies may very well provide information about the mechanisms associated with the preliminary gender differences in exposure and PTSD observed to date.

Recently, Breslau and colleagues (1998) found that assaultive violence (which included rape) induced the highest rate of PTSD of all the traumatic events measured. Yet the sudden and unexpected death of a loved one contributed the highest proportion of PTSD cases (31%) due to its high frequency in the population (60%). These researchers also found that PTSD persisted longer in women than in men; often persisted longer than 6 months (74%); and persisted longer when the traumatic event was directly rather than indirectly experienced. This study also found racial differences in the development of PTSD in that nonwhites were almost twice as likely to develop PTSD after exposure than were whites. These findings require continued study so that the mechanisms involved can be more fully understood.

Assessment of PTSD

Clinicians are increasingly recognizing that a sizable number of their clinical patients have experienced traumatic events and that the care of some patients is complicated by the presence of PTSD. Accordingly, there has been great interest among clinicians in the proper assessment and evaluation of patients with PTSD. Clearly, PTSD is assessed for many different purposes, and the goals of a particular assessment can determine the approach selected by the professional. Clinicians may wish to use a structured assessment as part of a diagnostic workup that includes a differential diagnosis and treatment planning. They may also be involved in forensic evaluations in which diagnostic accuracy is of utmost importance. Researchers may be interested in the frequency of occurrence of PTSD and the risk factors and complications associated with it (as in epidemiological studies). Moreover, researchers may be interested in high levels of diagnostic accuracy when studying biological and psychological parameters of the disorder, as in case-control studies. Each clinical and research situation requires a different solution depending on the assessment goals of the professional. For this reason, we present a general overview of the methods by which a clinician can evaluate the quality of available instruments.

The quality of psychological assessment is examined through the two psychometric characteristics of reliability and validity. Reliability is the consistency or replicability of test scores. Validity is the meaningfulness or accuracy inferences, interpretations, or decisions made on the basis of scores on tests or instruments. Test developers often report the consistency of tests over time (test-retest reliability), among different interviewers or raters (interrater reliability), or over the many items constituting a particular test (internal consistency). Reliability is reported for continuous measures as a simple correlation coefficient that can vary between 0.0 and 1.0. Reliability for dichotomous measures such as diagnostic interviews (indicating the presence or absence of a disorder) is often reported as a κ coefficient (Cohen 1960), which is also reported as 0.0–1.0 and is interpreted as the percentage agreement above chance.

Measures of validity include content validity, which represents the extent to which a test provides coverage of the domain of symptoms of a condition. The better the coverage of key symptoms, the better the content validity. If the measure of a disorder predicts something of interest or importance such as response to an intervention, it is said to have good criterion-related validity. Finally, if a measure is correlated with other measures of the same disorder it is said to have good construct validity.

Diagnostic instruments in the field of mental health are usually evaluated on the basis of their diagnostic utility, a type of criterion-related validity pertaining to a test's capacity to predict diagnostic status (Kraemer 1992). There are three steps in determining the diagnostic utility of a given instrument. First, a "gold standard" is selected. In psychological research, this is ordinarily a diagnosis made using a clinical interview, but it may also be a composite based on several sources of information. Second, both the gold standard and the newly developed test are administered to the experimental group of participants. Finally, a variety of cutoff scores are examined to determine their diagnostic utility or their ability to predict the diagnosis provided by the gold standard. Optimal cutoff scores for the test are those that predict the greatest number of cases and noncases from the original sample.

All measures of a psychological disorder are imperfect (Gerardi et al. 1989). Two measures of the error contained within a test are false positives and false negatives. A false positive occurs when a patient scores above the cutoff but does not have a true case of the disorder. A false negative occurs when a patient scores below the given cutoff yet in fact has a true case of the disorder. Diagnostic utility is often described in terms of a test's sensitivity and specificity. These are measures of a test's performance that take into account errors made in prediction. Sensitivity is the measure of a test's true positive rate, or the probability that those with the disorder will score above a given cutoff score. Specificity is the true negative rate of a test, or the probability that those without the disorder will score below the cutoff for the test. Sensitivity is low if the test yields too many false negatives, whereas specificity is low if the test yields too many false positives.

Selection of tests and diagnostic instruments should include an examination by the clinician of relevant data on their psychometric properties. Inspecting rates of false positives, false negatives, sensitivity, and specificity can also inform the clinician of how an instrument performs. Conclusions drawn in clinical assessment are most accurate if they take into account these limitations.

Efforts to diagnose and assess patients for the presence of PTSD can include a range of different approaches. These include structured diagnostic interviews for PTSD and related comorbidity, psychological tests and questionnaires, psychophysiologic measures, medical records, and the use of multiple informants on the patient's behavior and experiences. We have referred to this approach as a multimethod approach to the assessment of PTSD (Keane et al. 1987).

Structured Diagnostic Interviews

It is standard practice in clinical research to employ a structured diagnostic interview to ensure that all PTSD symptoms are reviewed in detail. Diagnostic interviews combine the virtues of defining precisely how a diagnosis was made with the use of interviews that have known psychometric properties (i.e., reliability and validity). The use of structured diagnostic interviews in the clinical setting is less common, with perhaps the single exception of clinical forensic practice, where it is strongly encouraged (Keane 1995). Nonetheless, the use of diagnostic interviews in clinical settings may well improve diagnostic accuracy and improve treatment planning (Litz and Weathers 1992). The use of broad-based diagnostic interviews that cover the range of high-frequency diagnoses will assist the clinician in that it will provide an evaluation not only of the target disorder but also the extent of clinical comorbidity that is present (Keane and Wolfe 1990; Weiss and Marmar 1997). Some of the available diagnostic interviews and their psychometric properties are described below.

Clinician-Administered PTSD Scale

Developed by the National Center for PTSD in Boston, the Clinician-Administered PTSD Scale (CAPS) was designed for use by trained, experienced clinicians (Blake et al. 1990). Consisting of 30 items, the CAPS assesses all 17 symptoms of PTSD as well as a range of the frequently observed associated features. Also contained in the CAPS are ratings for social and occupational functioning and an assessment of the validity of the responses by the patient. Like the PTSD-Interview and the Structured Interview for PTSD, the CAPS provides both dichotomous and continuous scores. Unique features of the CAPS are that it contains separate ratings for frequency and intensity of each symptom and that it possesses behaviorally anchored probe questions and scale values. Interviewers are trained to ask their own follow-up questions and to use their clinical judgment in arriving at the best ratings.

If administered completely (i.e., all questions regarding associated features, functional impairments, and validity ratings), the CAPS takes approximately an hour to complete. If only the diagnostic symptoms are assessed, the time for administration is cut in half.

Psychometric data on performance of the CAPS demonstrate unusual strength in identifying cases and noncases of PTSD. Across three clinicians and 60 separate male veteran subjects, Weathers and colleagues (1992) found test-retest correlations between 0.90 and 0.98. Internal consistency was equally impressive, with an α of 0.94 across all three primary symptom clusters. Correlations with other established measures of PTSD yielded strong evidence for the construct validity of the CAPS. The correlation of the CAPS with the Mississippi Scale was 0.91; correlation with the Keane PTSD Scale of the Minnesota Multiphasic Personality Inventory-2 (MMPI-2) was 0.77; and correlation with the Structured Clinical Interview for DSM (SCID) PTSD symptom score was 0.89. Correlations with a measure of antisocial personality disorder were low, as was predicted by the multitrait-multimethod study design.

Used as a continuous measure, the CAPS was found to have a sensitivity of 84%, specificity of 95%, efficiency of 89%, and κ of 0.78 against the SCID. Using the CAPS as a diagnostic measure, a κ of 0.72 was found compared with the SCID diagnosis. These findings establish that the CAPS is a sound measure of PTSD with excellent psychometric properties, whether it is used as a diagnostic or a continuous measure. Replications of these findings with male and female motor vehicle accident survivors (Blanchard et al. 1995) and with patients with serious mental illnesses of both sexes (Mueser et al. 1999) indicated the generalizability of these results across populations, races, and sexes. A recent publication carefully explicated nine different scoring algorithms for the CAPS and their implications for diagnostic accuracy, reliability, and validity coefficients (Weathers et al. 1999).

Structured Clinical Interview for DSM

The SCID (Spitzer et al. 1994) is the most widely used interview to assess Axis I and Axis II psychiatric disorders. It consists of separate modules for the most common diagnostic categories. Although the full SCID can be time consuming to administer, it does provide information across a broad range of clinical conditions. In many clinical settings, the SCID is used to systematically assess only the most frequently encountered conditions. This is economical in terms of time and still provides an examination across key conditions. For use in a trauma clinic, it is recommended that the anxiety disorder, affective disorder, and substance abuse disorder modules and the psychotic screen be employed. This provides a fairly comprehensive examination of the conditions that are frequently comorbid with PTSD and provides a systematic way to ensure that a patient does not show signs of psychoses—conditions that would require a different initial set of clinical interventions.

The PTSD module of the SCID appears to be both clinically sensitive and reliable. Keane and colleagues (1998) examined the interrater reliability of the SCID by asking a second interviewer to listen to audio tapes of an initial interview. They found a κ of 0.68 and agreement across lifetime, current, and never PTSD of 78%. Similarly, in a sample of patients who were reinterviewed within a week by a different clinician, these researchers found a κ of 0.66 and diagnostic agreement of 78%.

The primary limitation of the SCID is that it permits only a dichotomous rating of a symptom (present or absent), placing clinicians in a forced-choice situation. Most clinicians agree that psychological symptoms occur in a dimensional rather than a dichotomous fashion, and so the SCID seems limited by the use of the present/absent scoring algorithm. Several options have evolved in the field as a result of this limitation. These are described later in this chapter.

Anxiety Disorders Interview Schedule–Revised

Developed by DiNardo and Barlow (1988), the Anxiety Disorders Interview Schedule–Revised (ADIS) is a structured diagnostic interview that focuses primarily on the anxiety and affective disorders. The ADIS uses a

Likert-type scaling procedure for symptoms and is thus capable of being analyzed in multiple ways to determine the extent to which a symptom is present or absent. Psychometric properties of the ADIS PTSD module have been assessed in two separate studies, with mixed results. In the first study (Blanchard et al. 1986), a small group of combat veterans were assessed by two independent interviewers; excellent sensitivity (1.0) and specificity (0.91) were found. In a community-based study (DiNardo et al. 1993), the results were less impressive and the hit rates were less stable.

PTSD-Interview

Watson and colleagues' (1991) PTSD-Interview yields both dichotomous and continuous scores. The authors report strong test-retest reliability (0.95) and internal consistency (α=0.92), as well as strong sensitivity (0.89), specificity (0.94), and κ (0.82) compared with the Diagnostic Interview Schedule (Robins et al. 1981).

The PTSD-Interview appears to have excellent psychometric properties but differs in administrative format from most other structured diagnostic clinical interviews. With the PTSD-Interview, patients are provided a copy of the scale to read along with the interviewer. From this copy of the scale, they are asked to give to the clinician their rating on the Likert scale for each of the symptoms. This format has much in common with self-report questionnaires, yet it deviates from the other diagnostic scales in that it does not allow clinicians to make ratings of their own and use their expertise and experience.

Structured Interview for PTSD

The Structured Interview for PTSD (SI-PTSD) was developed by Davidson and colleagues (1989). As with the PTSD-Interview, it also yields both dichotomous and continuous measures of PTSD symptoms. As a result, it appears to be a useful instrument for diagnosing PTSD and measuring symptom severity. Symptoms are rated by the clinician on five-point Likert scales, and the focus for the clinician is on symptom severity. It possesses initial probe questions and provides helpful follow-up questions to promote a more thorough understanding of the patient's symptom experiences. In a study of male combat veterans, the Davidson and colleagues found sensitivity of 0.96 and specificity of 0.80, suggesting sound performance.

PTSD Symptom Scale Interview

Developed by Foa and colleagues (1993), the PTSD Symptom Scale Interview (PSS-I) possesses many strong clinical features that warrant its consideration for clinical and research use. Consisting of the 17 criteria of the

PTSD diagnosis, the PSS-I uses Likert-type rating scales for each of the criterion symptoms. It can be scored as a continuous and dichotomous measure of PTSD and takes approximately 20 minutes for completion. Administering this measure to 118 women with sexual assault histories, Foa and colleagues (1993) found excellent interrater reliability, diagnostic sensitivity of 0.88, and specificity of 0.96. Test-retest reliability over 1 month was also reported to be strong.

The advantages of the PSS-I are its relative brevity, its promising psychometric properties, and its use of Likert rating scales that provide both a dichotomous and a continuous scoring routine. Another strength of this interview is its development and validation with sexual assault survivors, a population of great interest and importance clinically.

Self-Report PTSD Questionnaires

Several self-report measures have been developed as a time-efficient and cost-efficient method for obtaining information on PTSD symptoms. These measures enjoy widespread acceptance and use due to ease of administration and scoring, and they are also useful adjuncts to the structured diagnostic instruments. They can also be invaluable when used as screens for PTSD. These measures are most frequently used as continuous measures of PTSD, but specific cutoff scores can be used to arrive at a diagnosis of PTSD.

PTSD Checklist

Developed (as was the CAPS) by researchers at the National Center for PTSD in Boston, the PTSD Checklist (PCL) comes in two versions: one for civilians and the other for military personnel. The scale contains the 17 items of the DSM diagnostic criteria scored on a five-point Likert scale. Weathers and colleagues (1993) examined its psychometric properties and found excellent internal consistency ($\alpha = 0.97$), excellent test-retest reliability over a 2- to 3-day period (0.96), and strong correlations with other measures of PTSD. The association with the Mississippi Scale was 0.93, association with the Keane scale was 0.77, and association with the Impact of Event Scale was 0.90. Blanchard and colleagues (1996) used the PCL in their studies of motor vehicle accident victims and found that the correlation of the PCL with the CAPS was 0.93 and overall diagnostic efficiency was 0.90 compared with the CAPS. The properties of the PCL with other populations have yet to be reported in the literature.

Impact of Event Scale–Revised

Initially developed by Horowitz and colleagues (1979), the Impact of Event Scale (IES) was revised by Weiss and Marmar (1997) to incorporate the symptoms of hyperarousal for PTSD (criterion D). The original scale contained only reexperiencing symptoms and avoidance/numbing symptoms and needed to be revised to more closely parallel the diagnostic picture. Although the authors provided some preliminary data, more information is needed about the reliability and validity of the revision. The most frequently used measure of PTSD, the original IES possessed good psychometric properties. Similar studies with the revised instrument will ensure its continued use in clinics and research settings.

Mississippi Scale for Combat-Related PTSD

The Mississippi Scale (Keane et al. 1988) is a 35-item scale designed to measure combat-related PTSD. The items were selected from an initial pool of 200 items generated by experts to closely match the DSM-III criteria for the disorder. The Mississippi Scale has excellent psychometric properties, with an α of 0.94 and test-retest reliability of 0.97 over a 1-week interval. Using a cutoff score of 107, the Mississippi Scale had strong sensitivity (0.93) and specificity (0.89).

These results were replicated in an independent laboratory by McFall et al. (1990), who found that the Mississippi Scale was highly correlated with the SCID PTSD module. These findings suggest that the Mississippi Scale, widely used in clinical and research settings serving veterans, is a valuable self-report tool.

Keane PTSD Scale of the MMPI-2

Originally derived from the MMPI Form R, the Keane PTSD Scale now consists of 46 items empirically drawn from the MMPI-2 (Keane et al. 1984; Lyons et al. 1992). The original report on the scale indicated that the Keane PTSD Scale correctly classified some 82% of the 200 subjects in the study. Subsequent studies confirmed these findings in combat veteran populations (Watson et al. 1986).

In terms of reliability, Graham (1990) found the Keane PTSD Scale to have strong internal consistency (0.85–0.87) and test-retest reliability (0.86–0.89). Although only a few studies have been conducted to date on the Keane PTSD Scale in nonveteran populations, the data presented appear to be promising (Koretzky and Peck 1990). More research is needed in this area, especially in the area of forensic psychology, where the MMPI-2 is frequently employed because of its validity indexes.

Penn Inventory for Posttraumatic Stress

The Penn Inventory is a 26-item questionnaire developed by Hammerberg (1992). Its psychometric properties have been examined in multiple trauma populations, and its specificity is comparable to that of the Mississippi

Scale, whereas its sensitivity is only slightly lower. It has been used with accident victims, veterans, and general psychiatric patients. It has primarily been employed with samples of male patients.

Posttraumatic Diagnostic Scale

Developed by Foa and colleagues (1997), the Posttraumatic Diagnostic Scale (PTDS) is derived from the DSM criteria directly. The items of the PTDS map directly onto the DSM-IV criteria for PTSD, and thus the questionnaire is 17 questions long. The PTDS begins with a 12-question checklist to elucidate the traumatic events to which an individual might have been exposed. Next, the patient is asked to indicate which of the events experienced has bothered him or her the most in the past month. The patient then rates his or her reactions to the event at the time of its occurrence to determine if the event fits both criteria A1 and A2.

The patient then rates on a single four-point scale the intensity and frequency of each of the 17 symptoms of PTSD that he or she has experienced in the past 30 days. The final section of the scale asks for self-ratings of impairment across nine areas of life functioning. This scale was validated using several populations, including combat veterans, accident victims, sexual and nonsexual assault survivors, and persons who had experienced a range of other traumatic events.

The psychometric analyses proved to be exceptional. For internal consistency, the coefficient α was 0.92 overall; test-retest reliability for the diagnosis of PTSD over a 2- to 3-week interval was also high (κ=0.74). For symptom severity the test-retest correlation was 0.83. Compared with a SCID diagnosis of PTSD, a κ coefficient of 0.65 was obtained with 82% agreement; the sensitivity of the test was 0.89, and its specificity was 0.75. Clearly, this self-report scale functioned well in comparison to the clinician ratings obtained in the SCID. It is a useful self-report and screening device for measuring PTSD and its symptom components.

Los Angeles Symptom Checklist

Consisting of 43 items scored on Likert-type scales, the Los Angeles Symptom Checklist (LASC) has been extensively studied across different populations (males and females, adults and adolescents, various trauma types). King and colleagues (1995) examined the psychometric properties of the LASC and found it to possess high internal consistency (α values ranging from 0.88 to 0.95) and test-retest reliability over a 2-week interval (0.90 and 0.94). Its strengths include the various ways in which it can be scored (continuously or dichotomously) and its inclusion of a range of associated features, signs of distress, and functional problems. Using only the 17-item PTSD index, King and colleagues (1995) found sensitivity of

0.74, specificity of 0.77, and an overall hit rate of 76% compared with a SCID diagnosis.

The use of these self-report questionnaires in a wide range of clinical and research contexts seems well supported by the extant data. It is clear that they can be successfully employed to measure PTSD symptoms when administering a structured diagnostic interview is not feasible or practical. Many of the measures can be used interchangeably, as the findings appear to be robust for the minor variations in methods and approaches involved. In selecting a particular instrument the clinician is encouraged to examine the data for that instrument for the population on which it is to be employed. In so doing, the clinician is likely to maximize the accuracy and efficiency of the test employed.

Psychophysiologic Measures

Research on biologically based measures of PTSD has grown tremendously in the past 10 years. Findings suggest that PTSD alters a wide range of physiologic functions (Yehuda 1997) and may also affect structural components of the brain (Bremner et al. 1995). To date, these findings have not been subjected to rigorous psychometric testing (i.e., utility analyses) to determine the extent to which these deviations are predictive of PTSD and non-PTSD cases. The primary exception to this conclusion is in the area of psychophysiologic reactivity, which from the start examined diagnostic accuracy (e.g., Blanchard et al. 1982; Malloy et al. 1983; Pitman et al. 1987).

The findings in this area clearly point to the capacity of psychophysiologic indices to identify and classify cases of PTSD on the basis of reactivity to auditory-, audiovisual-, and imagery-based cues. Measures have included heart rate, blood pressure, skin conductance, and electromyography. Studies covered the range of trauma survivors and include motor vehicle accidents, combat veterans from available eras, female sexual assault survivors, and survivors of terrorism. In perhaps the largest study of its kind, Keane and colleagues (1998) examined the responses of over 1,000 combat veterans to audiovisual- and imagery-based cues of combat experiences. The results supported the presence of elevated psychophysiologic arousal and reactivity in the participants, more than two-thirds of whom were correctly classified as having or not having PTSD.

Clearly, psychophysiologic assessment is costly in terms of time, patient burden, and cost. Yet in cases where much is at stake, it might be helpful to employ this assessment strategy clinically (Prins et al. 1995). Widespread adoption of this method of assessment is not expected due to the costs, the expertise required, and the success of other economical methods of assessment such as the diagnostic interviews and the psychological tests that are available.

As more information is collected on measures of the hypothalamic-pituitary-adrenocorticotropic axis, it is indeed possible that this system and measures of it could be useful adjuncts to the diagnosis of PTSD. In particular, indexes of cortisol, norepinephrine, and their ratio appear ready for an intensive examination for their capacity to improve diagnostic hit rates for PTSD above and beyond the use of diagnostic interviews and psychological tests (Yehuda et al. 1995).

Monitoring Outcomes in PTSD Treatment

Since the growth of managed care in the 1990s, there has been an increased need for clinicians to monitor the effects of their treatment interventions. Whether the intervention is psychopharmacologic, psychological, or a combination of the two, the use of psychological tests or questionnaires that possess excellent psychometric properties is recommended. For example, Keane and Kaloupek (1982), using a single-subject design, presented the first empirical evidence that cognitive-behavioral treatments for PTSD had promise. In that study, we employed subjective units of distress (SUDS) (0–10 ratings) within treatment sessions to monitor changes in the presentation of traumatic memories in a prolonged-exposure treatment paradigm. Between sessions, we used the Spielberger State Anxiety Inventory to monitor levels of anxiety and distress throughout the course of the 19 treatment sessions.

Similarly, Fairbank and Keane (1982) treated combat veterans with PTSD using a multiple-baseline design across traumatic memories. Measures to monitor change included SUDS ratings as well as heart rate and skin conductance response. Systematic improvement was observed in the treatment of traumatic memories, and this was evidenced in changes in SUDS ratings, heart rate, and number of skin conductance responses. Although this form of monitoring is intensive, it suggests that the level of change transcends self-report into the physiologic domains and thus is a rigorous assessment of the impact of the treatment provided.

With the expanding emphasis on the provision of problem-focused treatments, the need for evaluation of the effectiveness of treatment to payers and patients, and the growing use of quality assurance to monitor care in behavioral health programming, there is a corresponding need for the use of psychometrically sound instrumentation. Psychological tests and questionnaires often possess many virtues, including test-retest reliability, internal consistency, and indicators of validity. Moreover, they frequently present normative information against which an individual's performance can be compared with either the general population or target populations of interest (Kraemer 1992). For all these reasons, psychological tests are strongly warranted for consideration when clinicians are considering tools to monitor the outcomes of their interventions.

At least since the appearance of DSM-III (American Psychiatric Association 1980), the zeitgeist for monitoring treatment outcome has focused on symptomatology. Specifying symptom-level targets for change was a major advance in the methodology of psychotherapy outcome research. This focus on the microcosmic level of analysis yielded considerable benefit to the field, but unfortunately was at the expense of broader, macrocosmic levels of evaluation. This trend has been modified in recent years. Today, outcomes are measured at the symptom level, the individual level, the system level (i.e., economic or cost analyses), and at the social or contextual level. All are important and all can provide valuable information for clinicians and patients alike.

Most clinicians are well versed in the use of measures of anxiety, depression, and psychotic behavior and broad measures of psychopathology. Many appropriate measures of these domains exist, and clinicians are encouraged to look for measures that are suitable for their particular circumstances and settings. Use of these measures at intervals (e.g., daily, weekly, monthly, quarterly) during the course of treatment will provide knowledge of the patient's status and communicate to the clinician the extent to which the patient is changing in the desired directions.

Still, clinicians are encouraged to adopt additional measures to monitor treatment progress. These measures might incorporate the use of the SF-36 Health Survey, a broad-based measure of functioning that is widely used in the health care industry. Complete with many different scales to measure components of functioning, the SF-36 is easily administered, is well tolerated by patients, and is quickly becoming a standard in the field (Ware 1999).

Other instruments are available to measure other domains of patient satisfaction and services satisfaction (Atkisson et al. 1999), as well as the dimensions of marital satisfaction and quality of life (e.g., Frisch 1993). Selection of the most appropriate measure of outcome is fundamentally a clinical decision, one that needs to rest with the provider in consultation with the patient.

Summary

Diagnosing, assessing, and monitoring outcomes in PTSD is a topic of growing interest and concern in the mental health field (Wilson 1998). Since the inclusion of PTSD in the diagnostic nomenclature of the American Psychiatric Association, there has been considerable progress in understanding and evaluating the psychological consequences of exposure to traumatic events. Conceptual models of PTSD assessment have evolved (Keane 1991), psychological tests have been developed (Foa et al. 1998; Norris and Riad 1997), diagnostic interviews have been validated (Davidson et al. 1989; Foa et al. 1993; Weathers et al. 1992), and subscales of existing tests have been created to assess PTSD: for example, the MMPI-2 (Keane et al.1984) and the Symptom Checklist–90 Revised (Saunders et al. 1990). We can rightly conclude that the assessment devices available to assess PTSD are comparable to or better than those available for any other disorder in DSM-IV. Multiple instruments have been developed to cover the range of needs of the clinician. The data on these instruments are nothing short of outstanding.

The assessment of PTSD in clinical settings focuses on more than the presence, absence, and severity of PTSD. A comprehensive assessment strategy would certainly gather information about an individual's family history, life context, symptoms, beliefs, strengths, weaknesses, support system, and coping abilities. This would assist in the development of an effective treatment plan for the patient. The primary purpose of this chapter is to examine the quality of a range of different instruments used to diagnose and assess PTSD. However, the comprehensive assessment of a patient needs to include indexes of social and occupational functioning. Finally, a satisfactory assessment ultimately relies on the clinical and interpersonal skills of the clinician, because many topics related to trauma are inherently difficult for the patient to disclose to others.

This chapter is not intended to be comprehensive in its review of the psychometric properties of all instruments available. The goal was to provide a heuristic structure that clinicians might employ when selecting a particular instrument for their clinical purposes. By carefully examining the psychometric properties of an instrument, the clinician can make an informed decision about the appropriateness of a particular instrument for the task at hand. Instruments that provide a full utility analysis (e.g., sensitivity, specificity, hit rate) for the clinician to examine do much to assist clinicians in making their final judgments. Furthermore, instruments that are developed and evaluated on multiple trauma populations, for both sexes, and with different racial, cultural, and age groups are highly desirable; these are objectives for future study.

References

American Psychiatric Association: Diagnostic and Statistical Manual of Mental Disorders, 3rd Edition. Washington, DC, American Psychiatric Association, 1980

American Psychiatric Association: Diagnostic and Statistical Manual of Mental Disorders, 4th Edition. Washington, DC, American Psychiatric Association, 1994

Atkisson CC, Greenfield TK: The UCSF Client Satisfaction Scales, in The Use of Psychological Testing for Treatment Planning and Outcomes Assessment, 2nd Edition. Edited by Maruish M. Hillsdale, NJ, Erlbaum, 1999

Blake DD, Weathers FW, Nagy LM, et al: A clinical rating scale for assessing current and lifetime PTSD: The CAPS-1. Behavior Therapist 18:187–188, 1990

Blanchard EB, Kolb LC, Pallmeyer TP, et al: A psychophysiological study of post traumatic stress disorder in Vietnam veterans. Psychiatr Q 54:220–229, 1982

Blanchard EB, Gerardi RJ, Kolb LC, et al: Utility of the Anxiety Disorders Interview Schedule (ADIS) in the diagnosis of the post-traumatic stress disorder in Vietnam veterans. Behav Res Ther 24:577–580, 1986

Blanchard EB, Hickling EJ, Taylor AE, et al: Effects of varying scoring rules of the Clinician-Administered PTSD Scale (CAPS) for the diagnosis of post-traumatic stress disorder in motor vehicle accident victims. Behav Res Ther 33:471–475, 1995

Blanchard EB, Jones-Alexander J, Buckley TC, et al: Psychometric properties of the PTSD checklist (PCL). Behav Res Ther 34:669–673, 1996

Bremner JD, Randall TM, Scott RA, et al: MRI-based measures of hippocampal volume in patients with PTSD. Am J Psychiatry 152:973–981, 1995

Breslau N, Davis GC, Andreski P, et al: Traumatic events and posttraumatic stress disorder in an urban population of young adults. Arch Gen Psychiatry 48:216–222, 1991

Breslau N, Kessler RC, Chilcoat HD, et al: Trauma and posttraumatic stress disorder in the community: the 1996 Detroit area survey of trauma. Arch Gen Psychiatry 55:626–632, 1998

Cohen J: A coefficient of agreement for nominal scales. Educational and Psychological Measurement 20:37–46, 1960

Davidson J, Smith R, Kudler H: Validity and reliability of the DSM-III criteria for posttraumatic stress disorder: experience with a structured interview. J Nerv Ment Dis 177:336–341, 1989

De Girolamo G, McFarlane AC: The epidemiology of PTSD: a comprehensive review of the international literature, in Ethnocultural Aspects of Posttraumatic Stress Disorder. Edited by Marsella A, Friedman M, Gerrity E, et al. Washington, DC, American Psychological Association, 1996

DiNardo P, Barlow D: Anxiety Disorders Interview Schedule—Revised. Albany, NY, Center for Phobia and Anxiety Disorders, 1988

DiNardo P, Moras K, Barlow D, et al: Reliability of DSM-III-R anxiety disorder categories using the ADIS-R. Arch Gen Psychiatry 50:251–256, 1993

Fairbank JA, Keane TM: Flooding for combat-related stress disorders: assessment of anxiety reduction across traumatic memories. Behavior Therapy 13:499–510, 1982

Foa EB, Riggs DS, Dancu CV, et al: Reliability and validity of a brief instrument for assessing post-traumatic stress disorder. J Trauma Stress 6:459–473, 1993

Foa EB, Cashman L, Jaycox L, et al: The validation of a self-report measure of post-traumatic stress disorder: the Posttraumatic Diagnostic Scale. Psychol Assess 9:445–451, 1997

Gerardi R, Keane TM, Penk WE: Utility: sensitivity and specificity in developing diagnostic tests of combat-related post-traumatic stress disorder (PTSD). J Clin Psychol 45:691–703, 1989

Graham J: MMPI-2: Assessing Personality and Psychopathology. New York, Oxford University Press, 1990

Green BL, Lindy JD, Grace MC, et al: Chronic posttraumatic stress disorder and diagnostic comorbidity in a disaster sample. J Nerv Ment Dis 180:760–766, 1992

Hammerberg M: Penn Inventory for Posttraumatic Stress Disorder: Psychometric properties. Psychol Assess 4:67–76, 1992

Horowitz MJ, Wilner N, Alvarez W: Impact of Event Scale: a measure of subjective distress. Psychosom Med 41:209–218, 1979

Keane TM: Guidelines for the forensic psychological assessment of PTSD claimants, in Post-Traumatic Stress Disorder in Litigation. Edited by Simon RI. Washington, DC, American Psychiatric Press, 1995, 99–115

Keane TM, Kaloupek DG: Imaginal flooding in the treatment of posttraumatic stress disorder. J Consult Clin Psychol 50:138–140, 1982

Keane TM, Wolfe J: Comorbidity in post-traumatic stress disorder: an analysis of community and clinical studies. Journal of Applied Social Psychology 20:1776–1788, 1990

Keane TM, Malloy PF, Fairbank JA: Empirical development of an MMPI subscale for the assessment of combat-related posttraumatic stress disorder. J Consult Clinical Psychol 52:888–891, 1984

Keane TM, Wolfe J, Taylor KL: Post-traumatic stress disorder: evidence for diagnostic validity and methods of psychological assessment. J Clin Psychol 43:32–43, 1987

Keane TM, Caddell JM, Taylor KL: Mississippi Scale for Combat-Related Posttraumatic Stress Disorder: three studies in reliability and validity. J Consult Clin Psychol 56:85–90, 1988

Keane TM, Kolb LC, Kaloupek DG, et al: Utility of psychophysiological measurement in the diagnosis of post-traumatic stress disorder: results from a Department of Veterans Affairs cooperative study. J Consult Clin Psychol 66:914–923, 1998

Keane TM, Weathers FW, Foa EB: Diagnosis and assessment, in Effective Treatments for PTSD. Edited by Foa EB, Keane TM, Friedman MJ. New York, Gulford, 2000, pp 18–36

Kessler RC, Sonnega A, Bromet E, et al: Posttraumatic stress disorder in the National Comorbidity Survey. Arch Gen Psychiatry 52:1048–1060, 1995

Kilpatrick D, Edmonds CN, Seymour AK: Rape in America: A Report to the Nation. Arlington, VA, National Victims Center, 1992

Kilpatrick D, Saunders B: Prevalence and Consequences of Child Victimization: Results From the National Survey of Adolescents. Washington, DC, National Institute of Justice, 1999

King LA, King DW, Leskin G, et al: The Los Angeles Symptom Checklist: a self-report measure of posttraumatic stress disorder. Assessment 2:1–17, 1995

Koretzky MB, Peck AH: Validation and cross-validation of the PTSD subscale of the MMPI with civilian trauma victims. J Clin Psychol 46:296–300, 1990

Kraemer HC: Evaluating medical tests: objective and quantitative guidelines. Newbury Park, CA, Sage Press, 1992

Lyons JA, Keane TM: Keane PTSD Scale: MMPI and MMPI-2 update. J Trauma Stress 5:111–117, 1992

Malloy PF, Fairbank JA, Keane TM: Validation of a multimethod assessment of posttraumatic stress disorders in Vietnam veterans. J Consult Clin Psychol 51(4):488–494, 1983

McFall ME, Smith DE, Mackay PW, et al: Reliability and validity of Mississippi Scale for Combat-Related Posttraumatic Stress Disorder. Psychol Assess 2:114–121, 1990

Mueser KT, Salyers M, Rosenberg SD, et al: Reliability of trauma and PTSD assessments in persons with severe mental illness. Paper in submission, 1999

Norris F: Epidemiology of trauma: frequency and impact of different potentially traumatic events on different demographic groups. J Consult Clin Psychol 60:409–418, 1992

Norris F, Riad J: Standardized self-report measures of civilian trauma and posttraumatic stress disorder, in Assessing Psychological Trauma and PTSD. Edited by Wilson J, Keane TM. New York, Guilford, 1997

Pitman RK, Orr SP, Forgue DF, et al: Psychophysiological assessment of posttraumatic stress disorder imagery in Vietnam combat veterans. Arch Gen Psychiatry 44:970–975, 1987

Prins A, Kaloupek DG, Keane TM: Psychophysiological evidence for autonomic arousal and startle in traumatized adult populations, in Neurobiological and Clinical Consequences of Stress: From Normal Adaptation of PTSD. Edited by Friedman MJ, Charney DS, Deutch AY. New York, Raven, 1995

Resnick HS, Kilpatrick DG, Dansky BS, et al: Prevalence of civilian trauma and posttraumatic stress disorder in a representative national sample of women. J Consult Clin Psychol 61:984–991, 1993

Robins LN, Helzer JE, Croughan JL, et al: National Institute of Mental Health diagnostic interview schedule: its history, characteristics, and validity. Arch Gen Psychiatry 38:381–389, 1981

Saunders BE, Arata CM, Kilpatrick DG: Development of a crime-related posttraumatic stress disorder scale for women within the Symptom Checklist–90 Revised. J Trauma Stress 3:439–448, 1990

Spitzer R, Williams J, Gibbon M, et al: Structured Clinical Interview for DSM-IV (SCID). New York, Biometrics Research Department, New York State Psychiatric Institute, 1994

Vrana S, Lauterbach D: Prevalence of traumatic events and post-traumatic psychological symptoms in a nonclinical sample of college students. J Trauma Stress 7:289–302, 1994

Ware J: The SF-36 Health Survey, in The Use of Psychological Testing for Treatment Planning and Outcomes Assessment, 2nd Edition. Edited by Maruish M. Hillsdale, NJ, Erlbaum, 1999

Watson CG, Kucala T, Manifold V: A cross-validation of the Keane and Penk MMPI scales as measures of post-traumatic stress disorder. J Clin Psychol 42:727–732, 1986

Watson C, Juba MP, Manifold V, et al: The PTSD interview: rationale, description, reliability, and concurrent validity of a DSM-III-based technique. J Clin Psychol 47:179–188, 1991

Weathers FW, Blake DD, Krinsley KE, et al: The Clinician-Administered PTSD Scale: reliability and construct validity. Paper presented at 26th annual convention of the Association for Advancement of Behavior Therapy, Boston, November 1992

Weathers FW, Litz BT, Herman DS, et al: The PTSD Checklist (PCL): reliability, validity, and diagnostic utility. Paper presented at the 9th annual meeting of the International Society for Traumatic Stress Studies, San Antonio, TX, October 1993

Weathers FW, Ruscio A, Keane TM: Psychometrics properties of nine scoring rules for the Clinician-Administered PTSD Scale (CAPS). Psychological Assessment 11:124–133, 1999

Weiss DS, Marmar CR: The Impact of Event Scale–Revised, in Assessing Trauma and Posttraumatic Stress Disorder: A Clinician's Handbook. Edited by Wilson JP, Keane TM. New York, Guilford, 1997, pp 399–411

Yehuda R: Sensitization of the hypothalamic-pituitary-adrenal axis in posttraumatic stress disorder. Ann N Y Acad Sci 821:57–75, 1997

Yehuda R, Giller E, Southwick S, et al: Hypothalamic-pituitary-adrenal alterations in PTSD, in Neurobiological and Clinical Adaptations to Stress: From Normal Adaptations to PTSD. Edited by Friedman M, Charney D, Deutch A. New York, Raven, 1995

3

Specialized Treatment for PTSD

Matching Survivors to the Appropriate Modality

Edna B. Foa, Ph.D.
Shawn P. Cahill, Ph.D.

Although many people experience the symptoms of posttraumatic stress disorder (PTSD) shortly after exposure to a traumatic event, most experience a natural decline in symptoms over the course of the following several months (e.g., Riggs et al. 1995; Rothbaum et al. 1992). However, a substantial minority of trauma survivors continue to experience significant symptoms for months (Riggs et al. 1995; Rothbaum et al. 1992) and even years after the traumatic event (Kessler et al. 1995). Thus, not everyone exposed to a traumatic event goes on to develop PTSD, and of those who develop acute PTSD, not everyone goes on to develop chronic PTSD.

In the past decade, several psychological treatments have been developed and evaluated for their efficacy in the treatment of PTSD. Among these treatments, the various forms of cognitive-behavioral therapy have received the greatest research attention and support for their efficacy. For this reason, the discussion in this chapter is confined to cognitive-behavioral interventions, which include prolonged exposure, stress inoculation training, cognitive processing therapy, cognitive therapy, and eye movement desensitization and reprocessing. As with the natural recovery from PTSD, most people treated with one of these therapies show improvement. However, not everyone recovers, and most individuals continue to experience at least some residual symptoms. Taking these observations as a starting point, the goal of this chapter is to discuss factors associated with successful recovery, whether natural recovery or therapist-aided recovery; the relative efficacy of the different forms of cognitive-behavior therapy; and factors related to successful outcome and to matching clients with appropriate interventions.

Failure to Recover From Trauma: The Natural History of PTSD

Two prospective studies, one involving female rape victims (Rothbaum et al. 1992) and the other involving male and female victims of nonsexual assault (Riggs et al. 1995), provide examples of the natural course of PTSD symptoms over time. In both studies, participants were interviewed shortly after the index assault and then were evaluated weekly during the subsequent 12 weeks. The results were quite consistent across the two studies. Both studies indicated high rates of PTSD symptoms shortly after the trauma. In the study by Rothbaum et al. (1992) (Figure 3–1), 94% of the subjects met full symptom criteria for PTSD at the initial assessment, occurring an average of 13 days after the assault. However, by the fourth assessment, approximately 35 days after the assault—the point at which participants could be diagnosed with PTSD according to the duration criteria of DSM-IV-TR (American Psychiatric Association 2000)—the incidence rate for PTSD was 65%. By the final assessment 3 months after the assault—the point at which PTSD present in a participant would be considered chronic—the incidence rate was 47%. Subsequent analyses revealed that subjects who had PTSD 3 months after the assault showed greater symptom severity at the initial assessment, improved at a slower rate, and essentially reached a plateau in their recovery about 6 weeks after the assault.

The study by Riggs et al. (1995) revealed a similar pattern for victims of nonsexual assaults, with two exceptions: the initial levels of PTSD symptoms were not as high among the victims of nonsexual assault as they had been among the rape victims, and women reported greater symptom severity than men. For example, at the initial assessment, 71% of the women and 50% of the men met full symptom criteria for PTSD. At the fourth assessment (approximately 1 month after the assault), the rates of PTSD were 42% for the women and 32% for the men. By the final assessment, 21% of the women, but none of the men, met criteria for chronic PTSD. Similar to the findings by Rothbaum et al. (1992), subjects who displayed chronic PTSD had greater symptom severity at the initial assessment and their course of recovery appeared to reach a plateau by the fourth assessment,

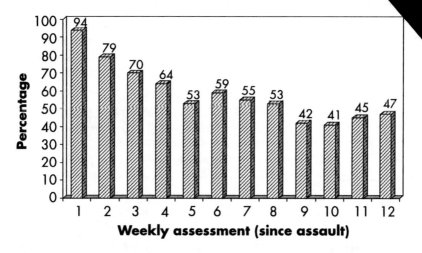

FIGURE 3–1. Percentage of victims meeting symptom criteria for PTSD after a recent rape.

Source. Reprinted from Rothbaum BO, Foa EB, Riggs DS, et al.: "A Prospective Examination of Post-Traumatic Stress Disorder in Rape Victims." *Journal of Traumatic Stress* 5:455–475, 1992. Copyright 1992 by the International Society for Traumatic Stress Studies. Used with permission.

whereas the group without chronic PTSD showed continuous improvement. It should be noted that sexual assault victims have shown a pattern of gradually declining symptom severity not only on measures of PTSD but also on measures of anxiety (Calhoun et al. 1982), depression (Atkeson et al. 1982; Rothbaum et al. 1992), and social adjustment (Resick et al. 1981).

These studies illustrate that most trauma victims show high levels of symptoms of PTSD, anxiety, and depression shortly after the traumatic event occurs, followed by gradual recovery during the subsequent 3 months. However, the studies also illustrate that for a significant minority of victims, PTSD becomes a chronic condition which, as Kessler et al. (1995) found, may last for years if left untreated.

Emotional Processing of a Trauma: Predictors of Recovery From PTSD

Foa and her colleagues have proposed that the development of PTSD after a traumatic event reflects a disruption of the normal emotional processing of the event (e.g., Foa 1993; Foa and Riggs 1993; Foa and Rothbaum 1998). Furthermore, Foa (1997) suggested that effective treatments decrease symptoms of PTSD by promoting engagement of the same psychological lie natural recovery.

ιotional processing theory (Foa and Kozak 1986),
ιmote recovery from anxiety disorders: emotional
feared stimuli (i.e., activation of the fear structure
er), habituation of the fear responses represented in
modification of the erroneous cognitions embedded
... structure. Foa and colleagues (e.g., Foa and Riggs 1993) hypothesized that the erroneous cognitions underlying PTSD involve the perceptions that the world is extremely dangerous and the self is totally
incompetent. This hypothesis has been supported in a recent study (Foa et
al. 1999b) that indicates that elevated perceptions of world-dangerousness
and self-incompetence distinguished individuals with PTSD from both
trauma victims without PTSD and nontraumatized individuals. According
to emotional processing theory, for a treatment of PTSD to be successful,
it should promote emotional engagement of the traumatic memories, facilitate habituation, and modify the erroneous cognitions underlying PTSD.
Evidence for each of these three suppositions is discussed below.

The Emotional Engagement Hypothesis

As discussed above, most trauma victims initially exhibit high levels of symptoms of PTSD, anxiety, and depression, which then gradually decline over
time. However, some individuals report dissociative experiences during or
shortly after a traumatic event, which have been found to be associated with
greater severity of PTSD symptoms later on (Cardena and Spiegel 1993;
Koopman et al. 1994). If high levels of dissociation are taken to indicate the
absence of emotional engagement, then the findings of these studies are consistent with Foa's (1997) hypothesis that just as emotional engagement is required for successful treatment of PTSD, it is also required for natural
recovery from a traumatic event. Accordingly, Gilboa-Shechtman and Foa
(2001) suggested that a peak in PTSD symptoms shortly after a traumatic
event signifies high initial emotional engagement and therefore should be associated with good recovery later on. In contrast, a delayed peak in PTSD
symptoms is thought to reflect low emotional engagement and therefore
should be associated with poor recovery later on.

To examine whether an early peak in PTSD symptoms is associated
with better recovery than a delayed peak, Gilboa-Shechtman and Foa
(2001) reanalyzed data from the study by Rothbaum et al. (1992) on the
natural course of symptoms following rape, utilizing individual growth
modeling (Willet and Sayer 1994). This technique assumes that everyone
displays a common reaction pattern (growth model), although individuals
may differ in the temporal characteristics (growth parameters) of their

reactions. The variables used to predict PTSD and depression 14 weeks after the traumatic event were the magnitude of each person's initial reaction, the magnitude of the peak reaction, and the timing of the peak reaction (days since the traumatic event). The results revealed that the magnitude of the *peak* reaction was a stronger predictor of outcome than was the magnitude of the *initial* reaction. In addition, the magnitude and timing of the peak reaction were better predictors of the rate of improvement than was the magnitude of the initial reaction. Consistent with this hypothesis, individuals whose peak response occurred within 2 weeks of the event exhibited less PTSD and depression 14 weeks after the trauma than did those whose peak response occurred between 2 and 6 weeks after the trauma.

Creamer et al. (1992) advanced a somewhat similar model of post-trauma processing, proposing that intrusions occur when a traumatic memory network has been activated. The immediate consequences of activating the traumatic memory network, they hypothesized, are increased symptoms of emotional distress and avoidance behavior. However, because intrusions are conceptualized as representing efforts to process the event, the model predicts that high levels of intrusions at one point in time should be predictive of lower intrusions at a later point in time. This model was tested with trauma victims who were present in an office building when a gunman killed eight people and who were assessed 4, 8, and 14 months after the trauma. As predicted, there was a significant relationship between intrusions and avoidance at each of the evaluations. Also as predicted, the severity of intrusions at the 4-month assessment was negatively associated with general distress at 8 months. Similarly, severity of intrusions at the 8-month assessment was negatively associated with general distress at the 14-month assessment. These results converge with those of Gilboa-Shechtman and Foa (2001), and both studies provide support for the view that early PTSD symptoms reflect emotional engagement, which in turn promotes recovery.

If the same processes underlie both natural recovery and improvement after treatment, then just as dissociation during or shortly after the trauma interferes with emotional engagement and thereby inhibits recovery, the absence of emotional engagement during exposure therapy should hinder the efficacy of a treatment aimed at reducing the severity of PTSD symptoms. To examine this hypothesis, Foa et al. (1995b) measured the magnitude of facial expressions of fear during the first exposure therapy session and correlated it with treatment outcome. The results revealed that, as would be expected, pretreatment levels of PTSD were associated with greater facial expression of fear (i.e., greater emotional engagement) during treatment and that high facial fear expression, in turn, was associated with greater improvement. Interestingly, high levels of pretreatment anger were associated with reduced facial fear expression during exposure therapy as well as with reduced improvement. Thus, anger, like dissociation, appears to dampen emotional engagement during exposure therapy, which in turn reduces treatment efficacy.

The Habituation Hypothesis

Although emotional engagement appears to be necessary for recovery, emotional processing theory posits that emotional engagement by itself may not be sufficient. A second important process is habituation, the gradual reduction across successive exposure sessions of the amount of fear elicited by the traumatic memory. Utilizing cluster analysis, Jaycox et al. (1997) identified three different patterns of response during imaginal exposure for PTSD, as measured by subjective units of distress (SUDS) taken during patients' recounting of their traumatic event. Patients in the first cluster showed high levels of anxiety during the first session, followed by a gradual decline over the next five sessions (high initial engagement and subsequent habituation). Patients in the second cluster also showed high levels of anxiety during the first session but showed little decline of anxiety in subsequent sessions (high initial engagement without subsequent habituation). Patients in the third cluster showed substantially less initial activation of fear, which did not decrease over the course of treatment (low initial engagement without subsequent habituation). Patients who showed both engagement and habituation had significantly more improvement after treatment than either those who showed engagement without habituation or those who showed neither engagement nor habituation. Thus, the results of this study support both the emotional engagement and the habituation hypothesis.

The Cognitive Modification Hypothesis

Several trauma theorists have proposed that exposure to trauma changes a person's thoughts and beliefs, particularly as they relate to the safety of the world, trustworthiness of others, and personal competence (e.g., Ehlers and Clark 2000; Foa and Riggs 1993; Janoff-Bulman 1989, 1992; McCann and Pearlman 1990). One method that has been adopted to assess cognitions associated with traumatic events is the use of questionnaires. For example, Janoff-Bulman (1989, 1992) developed the World Assumptions Scale (WAS) to assess perceived self-worth and benevolence of the world, and Resick et al. (1991) developed the Personal Beliefs and Reactions Scales (PBRS). Janoff-Bulman (1989) found that the WAS discriminated between trauma victims and nonvictims. As noted above, however, not all individuals exposed to trauma develop chronic PTSD, and it stands to reason that only those who do not recover exhibit dysfunctional cognition. This hypothesis was examined in the study by Foa et al. (1999b) mentioned above. In this study, Foa and her colleagues compared the cognitions of trauma victims with PTSD to those of trauma victims without PTSD and to nontraumatized individuals using the WAS, PBRS, and their newly developed Posttraumatic Cognitions Inventory (PTCI). As hypothesized, individuals with PTSD showed elevated perceptions of the world as dangerous, low self-worth, and high self-blame compared with the other two groups. Also supportive of the hypothesis that dysfunctional cognitions about the world and self underlie PTSD is the finding that trauma victims who did not have PTSD did not differ from nontraumatized individuals. At present there are not adequate longitudinal data on these measures to determine whether cognitive changes correspond to changes in symptom patterns over the natural course of recovery from PTSD. However, there are some data suggesting that each of these measures may be sensitive to cognitive-behavioral interventions for PTSD (Foa 1997; Resick and Schnicke 1992; Tolin and Foa 1999).

A second method to assess cognitions in response to trauma and how they change over time is content analysis of narratives of traumatic event. Amir et al. (1998) examined the degree of articulation or complexity of narratives from sexual assault survivors. Results indicated that a greater degree of articulation of narratives obtained shortly after the assault (within 2 weeks) was associated with less anxiety shortly after the assault and with less severe PTSD symptoms 12 weeks after the assault. In a study that examined narrative changes over the course of exposure therapy, Foa et al. (1995a) found that narratives obtained at the end of treatment were characterized by a greater percentage of organized thoughts, increased use of words denoting thoughts and feelings, and decreased references to specific actions or dialogue that occurred during the target event. Correlational analyses indicated that a reduction of fragmentation in the narratives was associated with a decrease in anxiety and that an increase in organization was associated with a decrease in depression. Thus, both of these studies suggest that the processes involved in the organization and articulation of the traumatic memories are implicated in both natural recovery and recovery via treatment.

Cognitive-Behavioral Treatment of Chronic PTSD

There is now accumulating evidence for the efficacy of a number of cognitive-behavioral treatments for chronic PTSD. For example, there is now little disagreement that prolonged exposure and stress inoculation training (SIT) are effective treatments for PTSD. Although they have not yet been as well researched, variations of cognitive therapy, including cognitive restructuring and cognitive processing therapy (CPT), as well as variants of eye movement desensitization and reprocessing (EMDR) show great promise. Several reviews are available that summarize the basic efficacy literature for these treatments (e.g., Foa and Meadows 1997; Hembree and Foa 2000). Each of the four treatments is briefly described below, and the efficacy of each treatment is illustrated by discussing some studies.

Exposure Therapy

The notion that trauma treatments need to incorporate some form of exposure to the traumatic memory has a long history in psychology and psychiatry (e.g., Fenichel 1945). At present, this idea is embedded in exposure therapy. Exposure therapy is a set of interventions aimed at helping patients to confront their feared objects, situations, memories, and images. With PTSD, exposure programs typically consist of imaginal exposure (i.e., repeated emotional recounting of the traumatic memory) and in vivo exposure (i.e., repeated confrontation with trauma-related situations and objects that evoke unrealistic anxiety). The goal of this intervention is to help the patient emotionally process the trauma by vividly imagining the event and describing it aloud, including thoughts and feelings that had occurred during the trauma. In vivo exposure helps the processing of the trauma by instructing the patient to confront situations, places, or activities that trigger trauma-related fear and anxiety. The patient is instructed to remain in the anxiety-provoking situation until his or her fear declines (i.e., is habituated) by a significant amount. The rationale for exposure therapy for PTSD is that the avoidance of trauma-related memories and reminders prevalent in individuals with PTSD interferes with the emotional processing of the traumatic event and thus with recovery.

How does exposure therapy ameliorate PTSD? First, repeated imaginal reliving of the trauma and in vivo exposure promote habituation or reduction of the anxiety associated with trauma memory. This allows patients to discover that anxiety diminishes even without avoidance or escape. Second, reliving the trauma in the presence of an empathic therapist helps patients realize that thinking about the trauma is not at all dangerous. Third, repeated reliving of the trauma helps to decrease generalization of the trauma-related fear by promoting differentiation between the traumatic event and other somewhat similar, but safe, situations. The patient comes to see the trauma as a specific event rather than as a representation of the "dangerous world." Fourth, exposure to, rather than avoidance of trauma-related fears and memories helps to change the patients' view that having PTSD symptoms represents incompetence and weakness, as exposure promotes a strong sense of mastery.

Stress Inoculation Training

Among the various anxiety management programs, SIT (Meichenbaum 1974) has been the one most researched with PTSD. In SIT, patients are provided with techniques that they can use to manage and reduce their anxiety when it occurs. These techniques typically include breathing and relaxation training, cognitive restructuring, guided (task-enhancing) self-dialogue, assertiveness training, role playing, covert modeling, and thought stopping. Veronen and Kilpatrick (1983) adapted Meichenbaum's SIT for use with rape victims.

The theoretical model put forward by Veronen and Kilpatrick (1983) in their SIT program for rape victims is based on social-learning theory. The theory posits that a traumatic event evokes emotional, cognitive, and behavioral fear responses and that cognitive appraisals and attributions mediate these responses. Through classical conditioning, neutral stimuli (e.g., places, people, hair or eye color, certain activities, time of day) that are associated with the traumatic event acquire the power to provoke fear and anxiety. These neutral situations are subsequently avoided or escaped to decrease the anxiety they provoke, and the reduction in anxiety in turn reinforces these avoidance or escape responses. Treatment therefore aims to teach patients skills that they can use to manage (and decrease) rape-related fear and anxiety. Veronen and Kilpatrick's adaptation of SIT for rape survivors included education about trauma and PTSD, deep muscle relaxation, breathing exercises, role playing, covert modeling, thought stopping, and guided self-dialogue. Patients are explicitly instructed to use these skills when confronted with situations or activities that triggered rape-related anxiety and fear.

Cognitive Therapy

The theory underlying cognitive therapy posits that individuals have particular ways of thinking about the world, other people, and themselves (e.g., Beck 1976; Beck et al. 1985). These patterns of thinking influence the manner in which individuals interpret events, and it is the interpretation rather than events themselves that are responsible for the emotions evoked by the events. Thus, when neutral events are interpreted as being threatening, they give rise to pathological emotions, including anxiety, depression, anger, or guilt. In their adaptation of cognitive therapy theory to PTSD, Ehlers and Clark (2000) suggested that the core cognitive distortion underlying PTSD is the interpretation of the reexperiencing of symptoms of PTSD as threatening.

The goal of cognitive therapy for PTSD is to teach patients to recognize their trauma-related irrational or dysfunctional cognitions that lead to negative emotions. The patients also learn to challenge these cognitions (thoughts or beliefs) in a logical, evidence-based manner. The therapist helps the patient weigh all of the alternative interpretations of target events and to determine whether the belief is helpful and accurately reflects reality, and if not, to replace or modify it.

Eye Movement Desensitization and Reprocessing

Eye movement desensitization and reprocessing (EMDR) (Shapiro 1989, 1995) is a therapeutic approach that has generated much interest among trauma therapists and researchers. In EMDR, the therapist asks the patient to generate images, thoughts, and feelings about the trauma, to evaluate their aversive qualities, and to make alternative cognitive appraisals of the trauma or their behavior during it. As the patient at first focuses on the distressing images and thoughts, and later focuses on the alternative cognition, the therapist elicits rapid lateral eye movements by instructing the patient to visually track the therapist's finger as it is rapidly moved back and forth in front of the patient's face.

Originally, Shapiro (1991) regarded the lateral eye movements as essential to the processing of the traumatic memory, asserting that they reverse the neural blockage induced by the traumatic event. However, the assertion about the cardinal role of the rapid eye movements component of the treatment has not been supported by dismantling studies (e.g., Boudewyns and Hyer 1996; Pitman et al. 1996; Renfrey and Spates 1994).

Outcome Research

Many well-controlled studies have documented the efficacy and efficiency of exposure therapy in reducing PTSD and related pathology such as depression and anxiety (c.f. Foa and Rothbaum 1998). Keane et al. (1989) and Cooper and Clum (1989) found that veterans with PTSD treated with imaginal exposure (which they termed "imaginal flooding") improved relative to control subjects on the waiting list and those given standard treatment, although the magnitude of improvement was moderate. Exposure treatment has also been found to be quite effective with rape-related PTSD. Foa et al. (1991) compared the efficacy of nine sessions of prolonged (imaginal and in vivo) exposure, SIT, or supportive counseling with a waiting list control group. Participants were female rape victims with chronic PTSD. After treatment, patients who received either exposure therapy or SIT showed significant improvement from pretreatment evaluation, whereas those who received supportive counseling or were placed on the waiting list did not. The SIT group showed the most improvement on PTSD symptoms immediately after treatment. By the 3-month follow-up, however, the prolonged exposure group scored better than the other groups on symptoms of PTSD, depression, and anxiety. In a second study, using a modified prolonged-exposure program, Foa et al. (1999a) treated female victims of rape and nonsexual assault with prolonged exposure alone, SIT alone, or the combination of prolonged exposure and SIT. All treatment groups showed substantial reductions in PTSD severity and depression, whereas the waiting-list control group did not. Furthermore, on several indices of treatment outcome, exposure alone was superior to SIT and prolonged exposure and SIT combined (Figure 3–2).

In a third, ongoing study of female assault victims with chronic PTSD, Foa and colleagues (discussed in Foa and Dancu 1999) found that 9 or 12 sessions (determined by the rate of improvement in self-reported PTSD symptoms) of exposure alone and exposure with cognitive restructuring effected large and equal improvements on symptoms of PTSD and depression. Based on results from the 96 women who completed the study, exposure alone seems to be a more efficient program than exposure plus cognitive restructuring: 57% of women in the exposure-alone group have been able to end therapy at 9 sessions by meeting the success criterion of at least 70% improvement in PTSD symptoms; in contrast, only 23% in the combined group met this criteria after 9 sessions.

Resick and colleagues developed a program they called cognitive processing therapy (CPT) (e.g., Resick and Schnicke 1992, 1993), which addresses specific concerns and symptoms of rape victims with chronic PTSD. A cognitive therapy component of this treatment aims at teaching patients to identify and modify distorted beliefs that commonly result from rape, focusing on issues of safety, trust, esteem, and intimacy. CPT also includes an exposure component that consists of writing a detailed account of the rape and reading it repeatedly. Treating rape victims in groups, Resick and Schnicke (1992) reported significantly greater reduction in PTSD symptoms and in depression after CPT compared with a naturally occurring waiting-list control group. At both posttreatment and 6-month follow-up evaluations, none of the women treated with CPT met diagnostic criteria for PTSD. Resick and colleagues are currently conducting a study comparing the efficacy of 12 sessions of individually administered CPT with 9 sessions of exposure therapy alone for rape victims with PTSD. Preliminary results based on 45 participants indicated that both treatments are highly and equally effective (Foa 1999).

Other recent investigations of PTSD treatment have included patients

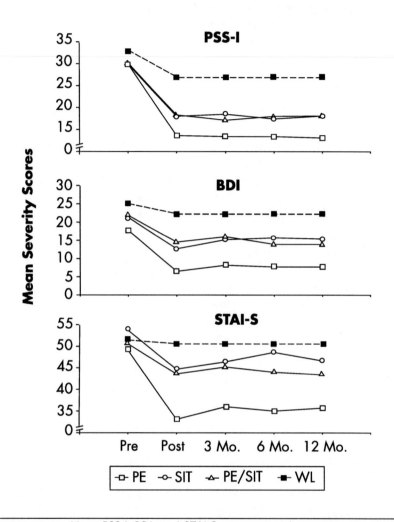

FIGURE 3–2. Mean PSS-I, BDI, and STAI-S scores at each assessment point for the four conditions (intent-to-treat sample, last value carried forward). Dashed lines indicate absence of follow-up data for WL participants. PSS-I = Posttraumatic Stress Disorder Symptom Scale-Interview; BDI=Beck Depression Inventory; STAI-S= State-Trait Anxiety Inventory–State Subscale; Pre=preassessment; Post= postassessment; Mo=months; PE=prolonged exposure; SIT=stress inoculation training; WL=waiting-list control.

Source. Reprinted from Foa EB, Dancu CV, Hembree EA, et al.: "A Comparison of Exposure Therapy, Stress Inoculation Training, and Their Combination for Reducing Posttraumatic Stress Disorder in Female Assault Victims." *Journal of Consulting and Clinical Psychology* 67:194–200, 1999. Copyright 1999 by the American Psychological Association. Used with permission.

whose PTSD resulted from a variety of traumas such as motor vehicle accidents, disasters, and childhood sexual abuse. Most of these studies have produced findings similar to those found in female assault victims. For example, Marks et al. (1998) conducted a study with patients diagnosed with chronic PTSD from a variety of traumas comparing exposure alone, cognitive restructuring alone, combined exposure and cognitive restructuring, and relaxation training. At the completion of treatment, prolonged exposure, cognitive restructuring, and the combination of prolonged exposure and cognitive restructuring were equally effective and were superior to relaxation training. Visual inspection of the data at the 6-month follow-up suggested a slight advantage for the groups that received exposure in comparison to those who received cognitive therapy alone. Tarrier et al. (1999) compared imaginal exposure (without in vivo exposure) to cognitive therapy in a sample of patients with PTSD resulting mostly from criminal victimization and motor vehicle accidents. The two treatments were found to be equally effective in ameliorating PTSD severity. However, the effects of both treatments were considerably more modest than those reported in previous studies of either treatment, raising questions about the manner in which the interventions were delivered.

Although a number of studies have evaluated the efficacy of eye movement desensitization and reprocessing (EMDR), most have not been well controlled. Some of the shortcomings of the studies are absence of blind, independent evaluators; lack of a pretreatment PTSD diagnosis via a valid assessment measure; and reliance on self-report measures for the main outcome variables. The general picture emerging from these studies is that EMDR is more effective than no treatment (i.e., waiting list control subjects). In a small study of EMDR (but the best controlled of the studied conducted to date), Rothbaum (1997) randomized 18 female rape victims with PTSD to either four sessions of EMDR or a waiting list. At posttreatment assessment, 90% of EMDR patients (compared with 12% of no-treatment patients) no longer met criteria for PTSD, and the effect size for the EMDR group was large. Treatment gains were found to be maintained at a 3-month follow-up assessment. In another study with a much larger sample (80 trauma victims, only 46% of whom met criteria for PTSD) and relying on self-report measures, Wilson et al. (1995) found that three sessions of EMDR significantly reduced PTSD severity, anxiety, and general distress compared with subjects on the waiting list. A 15-month follow-up study (Wilson et al. 1997) indicated that treatment gains had been maintained.

Results of studies that controlled for nonspecific treatment effects, such as the attention of a therapist and expectation of a positive outcome, yielded mixed results. Carlson et al. (1998) reported that in a group of veterans with PTSD, 12 sessions of EMDR produced greater improvement in PTSD symptoms than did 12 sessions of either relaxation training or standard care. However, these results were not consistent with those found in a study comparing EMDR, imagery habituation training, and applied muscle relaxation training with waiting list control subjects (Vaughan et al. 1994). All groups in this latter study improved significantly compared with the waiting list, and no differences emerged among the three treatment conditions.

Only one published study compared the efficacy of EMDR to a treatment of established efficacy for PTSD (Devilly and Spence 1999). In this study, patients were assigned to nine sessions of either EMDR or a cognitive-behavioral treatment package, called trauma treatment protocol (TTP), that consisted of a combination of prolonged imaginal exposure, SIT, and cognitive therapy. TTP patients showed significantly greater improvement on PTSD measures than did EMDR patients at both post-treatment and follow-up assessments. In addition, EMDR and TTP were rated as equally ("moderately") distressing. Taken together, the empirical studies on EMDR to date suggest that this treatment is effective for chronic PTSD, but more well-controlled studies are needed. Because the vast majority of the outcome studies on EMDR utilized primarily self-report measures, the hypothesis that the benefit of EMDR is due to non-specific treatment effects cannot be ruled out. Also, because EMDR incorporates repeated brief imaginal exposure and dismantling studies have generally failed to find evidence for an effect of eye movements, the hypothesis that the benefits of EMDR is due to exposure cannot be ruled out at this time either.

In summary, as noted earlier, many studies have indicated that exposure therapy is a very effective and efficient treatment for PTSD after a variety of traumas. SIT has also been found to be effective, but the evidence comes exclusively from studies on female assault victims, and the generalizability of the results to other populations is unknown. Cognitive therapy and EMDR are promising, but better-controlled studies are needed for a firm conclusion.

General Predictors of Treatment Outcome

In their study comparing prolonged exposure and cognitive therapy, Tarrier et al. (1999) reported that 12 of their 62 subjects who completed treatment showed an increase in PTSD scores from their pretreatment to their posttreatment assessments. Compared with those who improved with treatment, the patients who deteriorated during treatment perceived the treatments as less credible, were rated as being less motivated for treatment by their therapists, and, not surprisingly, attended fewer therapy sessions. Taylor et al. (in press) investigated predictors of treatment outcome and treatment completion among a group of 34 motor vehicle accident victims with PTSD. Their intervention was a multicomponent cognitive-behavioral treatment that included education, applied relaxation, cognitive restructuring, and imaginal and in vivo exposure. Consistent with the findings of Tarrier et al. (1999), Taylor et al. found that individuals who showed an increase in PTSD over the course of treatment had attended fewer therapy sessions. They also found that deterioration during treatment was associated with higher levels of stressful events not related to the index trauma occurring during the course of treatment, such as being fired from a job, the breakup of a romantic relationship, health problems, and financial problems.

In their analysis of variables associated with treatment completion, Taylor et al. (in press) found that those who did not complete treatment had a significantly larger number of comorbid psychiatric disorders, although the two groups did not differ in terms of the prevalence of any particular disorder. Noncompleters also had more severe PTSD, had higher levels of anxiety and depression, reported feeling more guilt about the accident, and perceived themselves as having less control over their lives. Finally, noncompleters were older, more frequently single, and had lower income than those who did complete treatment.

Predictors of Differential Treatment Outcome: Possible Matching Variables

As noted earlier in the chapter, there are a number of cognitive-behavioral therapies that have demonstrable efficacy for the treatment of PTSD. However, none of these treatments are effective with all patients. Therefore, it is entirely possible that treatments may be differentially effective for subgroups of individuals. If this is true, then it is important to be able to match treatments to patients, as such matching would be expected to improve overall efficacy of all treatments. To date, none of the published comparative treatment studies have investigated differential predictors of treatment outcome. Some information has emerged from an analysis of the data from the Foa et al. (1999a) study that compared SIT and prolonged exposure.

With regard to unique predictors of treatment outcome for prolonged exposure, we have found that a greater level of general anxiety at pretreatment assessment was associated with more severe PTSD symptoms at posttreatment assessment. However, high pretreatment severity of PTSD, depression, and poor social functioning were not related to treatment outcome for prolonged exposure. In contrast, poorer general social functioning before treatment predicted poorer social functioning and greater depression after treatment with SIT. Also, greater levels of pretreatment PTSD and depression predicted greater PTSD severity after treatment with SIT. These findings suggest that prolonged exposure may be more suitable for clients who initially present with poor social functioning, severe PTSD, or severe depression. In contrast, SIT may be more suitable for patients who present with high levels of general anxiety.

Summary and Conclusions

Empirical research suggests that several cognitive-behavioral therapies, including prolonged exposure, SIT, CPT, cognitive therapy, and EMDR, are effective with chronic PTSD, although a minority of patients still meet diagnostic criteria after treatment and many patients remain somewhat symptomatic. To date, prolonged exposure has received the most empirical support with the widest range of trauma populations. Also, compared with SIT, prolonged exposure affects a broader range of symptoms, reducing not only PTSD symptoms but also general anxiety and depression and increasing general functioning. Programs that combine prolonged exposure with other therapies (e.g., SIT, cognitive therapy) have not been found to be more effective than prolonged exposure alone, but more studies are needed on this issue.

Studies reviewed in this chapter suggest that when implementing cognitive-behavior therapy in general, and exposure therapy in particular, it is important to promote emotional engagement with the traumatic memory, as well as to promote conditions that will facilitate habituation of the anxiety associated with the traumatic memories. Finally, successful treatment of PTSD needs to change the erroneous cognitions that have been found to be associated with PTSD: that the world is entirely dangerous and the self is extremely incompetent.

The knowledge of how to treat chronic PTSD by far exceeds the knowledge about when treatment succeeds and when it fails. Not surprisingly, ongoing stress, low ability to function, noncompliance with treatment demands, and failure to complete the recommended number of treatment sessions are all factors that hinder good response to treatment. This means that patients who are most in need of treatment may be the ones who are unable to take advantage of the progress that has been made in the treatment of PTSD. The emphasis in the future should be on learning how to reach out to those who need treatment most and how to keep them in treatment once they seek help. If therapists pay attention to forming a strong alliance with patients, emphasize warmth and caring for patients, and are flexible in applying treatment, patient compliance and retention are likely to increase.

Very little is known about matching treatments to patients. The few available data suggest that exposure is the recommended treatment for patients with low general functioning at pretreatment assessment. Prolonged exposure appears to be the recommended treatment for individuals with high pretreatment levels of PTSD and/or depression. SIT, on the other hand, is recommended for patients with high pretreatment levels of general anxiety.

References

American Psychiatric Association: Diagnostic and Statistical Manual of Mental Disorders, 4th Edition, Text Revision. Washington, DC, American Psychiatric Association, 2000

Amir N, Stafford J, Freshman MS, et al: Relationship between trauma narratives and trauma pathology. J Trauma Stress 11:385–392, 1998

Atkeson BM, Calhoun KS, Resick PA, et al: Victims of rape: repeated assessment of depressive symptoms. J Consult Clin Psychol 50:95–102, 1982

Beck AT: Cognitive Therapy and the Emotional Disorders. New York, International Universities Press, 1976

Beck AT, Emory G, Greenberg RL: Anxiety Disorders and Phobias: A Cognitive Perspective. New York, Basic Books, 1985

Boudewyns PA, Hyer L: Eye movement desensitization and reprocessing (EMDR) as treatment for post-traumatic stress disorder (PTSD). Clinical Psychology and Psychotherapy 3:185–195, 1996

Calhoun KS, Atkeson BM, Resick PA: A longitudinal examination of fear reactions in victims of rape. Journal of Counseling Psychology 29:655–661, 1982

Cardena E, Spiegel D: Dissociative reactions to the San Francisco Bay Area Earthquake of 1989. Am J Psychiatry 150:474–478, 1993

Carlson JG, Chemtob CM, Rusnak K, et al: Eye movement desensitization and reprocessing for combat-related posttraumatic stress disorder. J Trauma Stress 11:3–24, 1998

Cooper NA, Clum GA: Imaginal flooding as a supplementary treatment for PTSD in combat veterans: a controlled study. Behavior Therapy 20:381–391, 1989

Creamer M, Burgess P, Pattison P: Reaction to trauma: a cognitive processing model. J Abnorm Psychol 101:425–459, 1992

Devilly GJ, Spence SH: The relative efficacy and treatment distress of EMDR and a cognitive-behavior trauma treatment protocol in the amelioration of post-traumatic stress disorder. J Anxiety Disord 13:131–157, 1999

Ehlers A, Clark DM: A cognitive model of posttraumatic stress disorder. Behav Res Ther 38(4):319–345, 2000

Fenichel O: The Psychoanalytic Theory of Neurosis. New York, WW Norton, 1945

Foa EB: Symptom patterns of assault-related posttraumatic stress disorder. Symposium entitled Manifestations of PTSD in Traumatized Populations—A Symptom-Level Analysis at the 101st American Psychological Association Annual Convention in Toronto, Canada, August 1993

Foa EB: Psychological processes related to recovery from a trauma and an effective treatment for PTSD. Ann N Y Acad Sci 821:410–424, 1997

Foa EB: Psychosocial treatment of posttraumatic stress disorder. Symposium entitled Focus on Post-Traumatic Stress Disorder presented at the International Consensus Group on Depression and Anxiety Consensus Meeting, Montecatinin, Italy, April 1999

Foa EB, Dancu CV: CBT of PTSD in female assault victims. Institute presented at the annual convention of the Association for Advancement of Behavior Therapy, Toronto, Ontario, Canada, November 1999

Foa EB, Kozak MJ: Emotional processing of fear: exposure to corrective information. Psychol Bull 99:20–35, 1986

Foa EB, Meadows EA: Psychosocial treatments for posttraumatic stress disorder: a critical review. Annu Rev Psychol 48:449–480, 1997

Foa EB, Riggs DS: Post-traumatic stress disorder in rape victims, in American Psychiatric Press Review of Psychiatry, Vol 12. Edited by Oldham JM, Riba MB, Tasman A. Washington, DC, American Psychiatric Press, 1993, pp 273–303

Foa EB, Rothbaum BO: Treating the Trauma of Rape: Cognitive-Behavioral Therapy for PTSD. New York, Guilford, 1998

Foa EB, Rothbaum BO, Riggs DS, et al: Treatment of posttraumatic stress disorder in rape victims: a comparison between cognitive-behavioral procedures and counseling. J Consult Clin Psychol 59:715–723, 1991

Foa EB, Molnar C, Cashman L: Change in rape narratives during exposure therapy for posttraumatic stress disorder. J Trauma Stress 8:675–690, 1995a

Foa EB, Riggs DS, Massie ED, et al: The impact of fear activation and anger on the efficacy of exposure treatment for posttraumatic stress disorder. Behavior Therapy 26:487–499, 1995b

Foa EB, Dancu CV, Hembree EA, et al: A comparison of exposure therapy, stress inoculation training, and their combination for reducing posttraumatic stress disorder in female assault victims. J Consult Clin Psychol 67:194–200, 1999a

Foa EB, Ehlers A, Clark DM, et al: The post-traumatic cognitions inventory (PTCI): development and validation. Psycological Assessment 11:303–314, 1999b

Gilboa-Shechtman E, Foa EB: Patterns of recovery following trauma: the use of individual analysis. J Abnorm Child Psychol 110:392–400, 2001

Hembree EA, Foa EB: Posttraumatic stress disorder: psychological factors and psychosocial interventions. J Clin Psychiatry 61(suppl 7):33–39, 2000

Janoff-Bulman R: Assumptive worlds and the stress of traumatic events: applications of the schema construct. Social Cognition 7:113–136, 1989

Janoff-Bulman R: Shattered Assumptions: Towards a New Psychology of Trauma. New York, Free Press, 1992

Jaycox LH, Foa EB, Morral AR: Influence of emotional engagement and habituation on exposure therapy for PTSD. J Consult Clin Psychol 66:185–192, 1998

Keane TM, Fairbank JA, Caddell JM, et al: Implosive (flooding) therapy reduces symptoms of PTSD in Vietnam combat veterans. Behavior Therapy 20:245–260, 1989

Kessler RC, Sonnega A, Bromet E, et al: Posttraumatic stress disorder in the National Comorbidity Survey. Arch Gen Psychiatry 52:1048–1060, 1995

Koopman C, Classen C, Spiegel DA: Predictors of posttraumatic stress symptoms among survivors of the Oakland/Berkeley, California, firestorm. Am J Psychiatry 151: 888–894, 1994

Marks I, Lovell K, Noshirvani H, et al: Treatment of posttraumatic stress disorder by exposure and/or cognitive restructuring. Arch Gen Psychiatry 55:317–325, 1998

McCann IL, Pearlman LA: Psychological Trauma and the Adult Survivor: Theory, Therapy, and Transformation. New York, Brunner/Mazel, 1990

Meichenbaum D: Cognitive Behavior Modification. Morristown, NJ, General Learning Press, 1974

Pitman RK, Orr SP, Altman B, et al: Emotional processing during eye movement desensitization and reprocessing therapy of Vietnam veterans with chronic posttraumatic stress disorder. Compr Psychiatry 37:419–429, 1996

Renfrey G, Spates CR: Eye movement desensitization: a partial dismantling study. J Behav Ther Exp Psychiatry 25:231–239, 1994

Resick PA, Schnicke MK: Cognitive processing therapy for sexual assault victims. J Consult Clin Psychol 60:748–756, 1992

Resick PA, Schnicke MK: Cognitive Processing Therapy for Rape Victims: A Treatment Manual. Newbury Park, CA, Sage, 1993

Resick PA, Calhoun KS, Atkeson BM, et al: Social adjustment in victims of sexual assault. J Consult Clin Psychol 49:705–712, 1981

Resick PA, Schnicke MK, Markway BG: The relationship between cognitive content and posttraumatic stress disorder. Paper presented at the annual meeting of the Association for Advancement of Behavior Therapy, New York, November 1991

Riggs DS, Rothbaum BO, Foa EB: A prospective examination of symptoms of posttraumatic stress disorder in victims of nonsexual assault. Journal of Interpersonal Violence 10:201–214, 1995

Rothbaum BO: A controlled study of eye movement desensitization and reprocessing in the treatment of posttraumatic stress disordered sexual assault victims. Bull Menninger Clin 61:317–334, 1997

Rothbaum BO, Foa EB, Riggs DS, et al: A prospective examination of post-traumatic stress disorder in rape victims. J Trauma Stress 5:455–475, 1992

Shapiro F: Efficacy of eye movement desensitization procedure in the treatment of traumatic memories. J Trauma Stress 2:199–223, 1989

Shapiro F: Eye movement desensitization and reprocessing procedure: from EMD to EMDR: a new treatment model for anxiety and related trauma. Behavior Therapist 14:133–135, 1991

Shapiro F: Eye Movement Desensitization and Reprocessing: Basic Principles, Protocols, and Procedures. New York, Guilford, 1995

Tarrier N, Pilgrim H, Sommerfield C, et al: A randomized trial of cognitive therapy and imaginal exposure in the treatment of chronic posttraumatic stress disorder. J Consult Clin Psychol 67:13–18, 1999

Taylor S, Fedoroff IC, Koch WJ: Posttraumatic stress disorder due to motor vehicle accidents: patterns and predictors of response to cognitive-behaviour therapy, in Road Accidents and the Mind: An In-Depth Study of Psychological Symptoms After Road Accidents. Edited by Blanchard EB, Hickerling EJ. Amsterdam, Elsevier (in press)

Tolin DF, Foa EB: Treatment of a police officer with PTSD using prolonged exposure. Behavior Therapy 30:527–538, 1999

Vaughan K, Armstrong MF, Gold R, et al: A trial of eye movement desensitization compared to image habituation training and applied relaxation in post-traumatic stress disorder. J Behav Ther Exp Psychiatry 25:283–291, 1994

Veronen LJ, Kilpatrick DG: Stress management for rape victims, in Stress Reduction and Prevention. Edited by Meichenbaum D, Jaremko ME. New York, Plenum, pp 341–374, 1983

Willet JB, Sayer AG: Using covariance structure analysis to detect correlates and predictors of individual change over time. Psychol Bull 116:363–381, 1994

Wilson SA, Becker LA, Tinker RH: Eye movement desensitization and reprocessing (EMDR) treatment for psychologically traumatized individuals. J Consult Clin Psychol 63:928–937, 1995

Wilson SA, Becker LA, Tinker RH: Fifteen-month follow-up of eye movement desensitization and reprocessing (EMDR) treatment for PTSD and psychological trauma. J Consult Clin Psychol 65:1047–1056, 1997

4

Rationale and Role for Medication in the Comprehensive Treatment of PTSD

Thomas A. Mellman, M.D.

Bridging Treatment to Emerging Knowledge of the Psychobiology of PTSD

Recently there appears to have been a marked increase in both the number of studies and clinical interest in the application of medication treatments for posttraumatic stress disorder (PTSD). This tendency may reflect other trends in the field and its current level of maturation. The period that preceded and immediately followed the official adoption of criterion-based diagnosis in DSM-III (American Psychiatric Association 1980) was beset by controversy and produced limited research. However, the field no longer seems to be stuck on certain basic issues. For example, it is now well accepted that both the experience of trauma and individual risk factors contribute to the development of PTSD in critical ways. High rates of psychiatric comorbidity are no longer viewed as a challenge to the validity of the disorder. A burgeoning number of neurobiological studies are generating new findings that are having an impact on the conceptual understanding of the nature of PTSD (see Chapter 2, in this volume). The various findings suggesting neurobiological alterations or abnormalities in PTSD also provide a basic justification for applying and empirically evaluating the therapeutic effects of pharmacologic agents. There continues to be some degree of dissociation, however, between the emerging knowledge base of the psychobiology of PTSD and the state of the art for medication treatment. However, this is not an unusual situation for psychiatry as well as other fields of medicine. The discovery of the first wave of psychotropic agents was largely serendipitous. Initial theories of the neurobiology underlying mood disorders and schizophrenia were derived from known mechanisms of action of drugs, rather than medications being developed based on known mechanisms of pathophysiology.

The principal rationale for most of the medication treatment that has currently been evaluated is the overlap (i.e., phenomenological similarity of certain features of the disorder and comorbidity) of PTSD with mood and other anxiety disorders. An important caveat to this approach is that biological findings between PTSD and these other conditions can be dissimilar or, as in the case of cortisol findings in PTSD and major depression, divergent. Nonetheless, there is evidence in studies of PTSD for dysregulations within the neurotransmitter systems that are the principal targets of "antidepressant" medications (i.e., serotonin and noradrenalin) (Southwick et al. 1997) as well as evidence supporting efficacy for these agents (see next section). The possible range of neurobiological systems that contribute to the pathogenesis of PTSD and are candidate targets for medication treatment has been thoroughly reviewed elsewhere (see Friedman and Southwick 1995). Disturbances in higher-order functions implicated in PTSD (e.g., conditioning and sensitization, memory consolidation, sleep regulation) might also be considered as a basis for formulating possible strategies for medication treatment and possibly other somatic interventions. At the present time there is evidence-based literature for the clinician to draw on to make decisions regarding prescribing medication for patients diagnosed with PTSD; this literature is reviewed below along with its limitations and additional rationales for consideration. It is expected and hoped that the current treatments being established—as well as the next wave of medications applied or developed for treating or preventing PTSD—will be validated by or evolve from an emerging understanding of the factors that contribute to the pathogenesis and maintenance of the disorder.

Overview of Evidence-Based Literature on Medication Treatment for PTSD

The standard for establishing efficacy for pharmacologic agents in the treatment of psychiatric disorders is the randomized controlled trial.

Because psychiatric symptoms frequently improve in response to "nonspecific" factors, the generally accepted standard—which furthermore is a criterion for U.S. Food and Drug Administration (FDA) approval for an indication—is demonstration of efficacy in comparison to treatment with placebo under blinded conditions. FDA approval of a medication treatment for the indication of PTSD was achieved substantially later than the establishment of numerous pharmacologic treatments for major depression and approval of a number of agents for other anxiety-disorder indications. Overall, the medication treatment literature for PTSD must be considered underdeveloped in comparison to that of other psychiatric disorders. That PTSD is among the most prevalent of psychiatric disorders and often has a persisting course (Kessler et al. 1995) justifies prioritizing treatment development. Additional justification for further research is that although the extent to which medication is utilized for PTSD in clinical practice is not known, it appears to be quite common.

The first application of medication treatment for PTSD (or for overlapping diagnostic terms predating DSM-III) documented in the literature was in open-label (i.e., not controlled) trials of the monoamine oxidase inhibitor (MAOI) phenelzine (Hogben and Cornfeld 1981). These positive reports were followed by several placebo-controlled trials of phenelzine or tricyclic antidepressant medications. Findings for the tricyclic antidepressants include demonstration of efficacy in comparison to placebo for imipramine and amitriptyline (Davidson et al. 1990; Frank et al. 1988). Therapeutic effects were noted specifically in the reexperiencing and heightened arousal symptom clusters. One of these studies included a comparison with phenelzine, which was also found to be efficacious compared with placebo, with therapeutic effects that exceeded those of imipramine, although not at a level of statistical significance (Frank et al. 1988). A review examining effect sizes for medication treatment studies of PTSD concluded that the largest treatment response has been observed for phenelzine (Friedman and Southwick 1995). Conclusions regarding the superiority of phenelzine must be tempered, however, by the existence of at least one study of phenelzine treatment with negative results (that may be limited by its design) (Shestatzky et al. 1988) and by a limited amount of data overall. It is also worth noting that the treatment effects of the tricyclic antidepressants, although previously considered to be of modest strength (Friedman et al. 1995), were nonetheless demonstrated in combat veterans treated in the setting of Veterans Administration (VA) medical centers. This observation is significant today, as findings from the recent studies of selective serotonin reuptake inhibitors (SSRIs) have not established that the efficacy of these agents extends to the subpopulation of male combat veterans.

There are also studies that are noteworthy for indicating where efficacy may not exist. For example, in one study (Braun et al. 1990), treatment with alprazolam did not significantly reduce PTSD symptom severity and was not differentiated from administration of placebo. This finding suggests that the response pattern of PTSD differs from those of panic disorder and generalized anxiety disorder. Among tricyclic antidepressants studied, more marginal effects were found for desipramine (Reist et al. 1989). Because desipramine is a more purely noradrenergic agent than the other tricyclics studied, the collective findings can be inferred to support a role for modulating serotoninergic neurotransmission in the pharmacotherapy of PTSD.

This support for the relevance of serotoninergic mechanisms presaged the recent advent of SSRIs as treatments for PTSD. In the 1990s, SSRIs emerged as popular agents for the treatment of depression and several anxiety disorders because of their broad spectrum of efficacy, relative safety, and ease of administration. It is also not surprising from this perspective that the SSRIs would be applied and tested for PTSD. The first published study to document efficacy compared with placebo treatment was for fluoxetine (van der Kolk et al. 1994). A more recent study reported by Conner et al. (1999) contrasts a number of the earlier studies of pharmacotherapy by demonstrating symptom reduction with fluoxetine compared with placebo in all of the DSM-IV-TR (American Psychiatric Association 2000) symptom clusters, including the cluster denoting numbing and avoidance. A large program documenting therapeutic effects for sertraline was published in a major medical journal (Brady et al. 2000) and supported the first FDA approval for PTSD as an implication. A similar multicenter trial documenting efficacy for paroxetine was recently published (Tucker et al. 2001). A caveat to the emergence of SSRIs as treatments for PTSD is that the populations in whom efficacy has been established are predominantly composed of adult women with PTSD related to sexual and nonsexual assault. The report of van der Kolk et al. (1994) included a subgroup of male combat veterans whose responses were negligible; furthermore, negative findings for SSRI treatment of combat veterans has been reported in meeting formats (Nagy et al. 1996). Nevertheless, for adult women with PTSD related to assault (who constitute a substantial proportion of the population with PTSD), evidence supporting efficacy of SSRI treatments (specifically fluoxetine and sertraline) is strong.

Given the open questions about population generalization and the limited number of agents tested in randomized controlled trials, observations from open-label evaluations seem to merit consideration with the caveat that any inferences must be considered tentative. Another open study suggests that the benefits of sertraline extend to PTSD comorbid with alcoholism (Brady et al. 1995). Nefazodone is a newer antidepressant with a distinct profile of serotoninergic effects that reduces awakenings and preserves rapid eye movement sleep in depression (Armitage et al. 1997) and has been found to improve symptoms of sleep disturbance and nightmares (Hidalgo et al. 1999; Mellman et al. 1999). Trazodone has also been reported to be useful for reducing sleep disturbances in PTSD patients (Ashford and Miller 1996). Anticonvulsants and mood stabilizers appear to be frequently utilized for PTSD. Rationales for this approach include the presence of bipolar-spectrum comorbidity, the targeting of impulsive aggression, and the possible relevance of kindling mechanisms to the progression of PTSD symptoms over time. Support for therapeutic effects of anticonvulsants on at least subgroups of PTSD symptoms is provided in reports of open-label treatment with carbamazepine (Lipper et al. 1986) and valproate (Fesler 1991). One line of research on the neurobiological underpinnings of PTSD suggested heightened reactivity of the central noradrenergic system (Southwick et al. 1997). There have been several observations, primarily of an anecdotal nature, of agents that suppress or block noradrenergic activity, reducing PTSD symptoms (Horrigan 1996; Kolb et al. 1984). Finally, although the current supporting evidence is limited, atypical neuroleptics are beginning to be considered for use in complex and otherwise refractory cases (Hamner 1996).

Limitations of Available Evidence-Based Literature

Limited Number of Randomized Trials That Test a Limited Number of Agents

Cited in the previous section are seven randomized controlled trials from the published literature on medication treatment for PTSD. Six of the studies featured medications categorized as antidepressants (tricyclics, MAOIs, and SSRIs). The other agent referred to, alprazolam, and another agent studied, inositol (Kaplan et al. 1996), were not found to be effective. The list of agents that have been supported by more anecdotal findings and observations or theory is more extensive. Thus, limiting prescribing to treatments supported by this reasonable standard for establishing efficacy (randomized controlled trials) would impose considerable constraint on the clinician.

Cases That Are Less Complicated Than Those Often Seen in Clinical Practice

The first wave of medication studies tended to emphasize combat veterans seeking treatment in VA or VA-affiliated settings. These studies support the existence of at least modest efficacy for tricyclic and MAOI antidepressants. It is unclear to what degree the veterans recruited 10 years ago for these studies are representative of the veterans currently presenting for treatment in VA settings for combat-related PTSD. Paradoxically, veteran subpopulations appear to be underrepresented in the recent wave of studies. This trend is partly a consequence of recent suggestions of treatment unresponsiveness in the VA-based veteran subpopulation (Nagy et al. 1996; van der Kolk et al. 1994) and the fact that a number of recent studies have been designed to establish efficacy to support an FDA-approved indication. Establishment of FDA approval is an important landmark for the field. The focus on this goal does have implications that affect the ability to generalize findings to subgroups of PTSD patients. For example, the necessity of establishing efficacy that is specific to the disorder in question is a rationale for placing limits on comorbid disorders. Such protocols typically require that certain comorbid disorders be clearly secondary in temporal onset and severity to PTSD and exclude other diagnoses. However, even in a community-based survey, it was found that PTSD was highly comorbid and that comorbid disorders were equally likely to precede or follow the onset of PTSD (Kessler et al. 1995). The presence of atypical psychotic or dissociative features would greatly diminish the likelihood of a patient participating in a contemporary medication trial. An additional requirement is that participants start taking no psychotropically active medications and receive monotherapy or placebo during the trial. Whether appropriate or not, it appears to be common for patients being treated for PTSD to receive combinations of medications, and such patients and their clinicians are often reluctant to discontinue existing regimens.

Absence of Published Studies of Controlled Trials of Combinations of Medication Treatments

Although the nature of prescription in clinical practice is not known, it is likely that many patients diagnosed with PTSD who are taking medication are prescribed more than one agent. Among the reasons that this is probably true are that in a significant number of cases a single agent may not be robustly effective for the spectrum of symptoms of PTSD and comorbid conditions that often present with the disorder. The degree to which the literature is underdeveloped and the establishment of few regimens as being definitively effective is also conducive to the practice of trying multiple agents. Although one can conceive of rationales for initiating different agents targeting subgroups of symptoms or comorbid presentations, data that support or argue against combination pharmacotherapy are limited. Whereas methods for augmenting response that are established or under investigation for mood disorders are largely unexplored with PTSD, the strategy of adding buspirone to antidepressant medication was recently reported to have been beneficial in an uncontrolled case series of PTSD patients (Hamner et al. 1997).

Absence of Published Studies Comparing or Combining Medication and Psychotherapeutic Treatments

It is likely that the modal treatment for PTSD is some combination of psychotherapy and medication. There is little if anything from the evidence-based literature to guide such treatment. In terms of extrapolating from the treatment literature of other psychiatric disorders, there does not appear to be any evidence from this literature that medication and psychotherapeutic treatment detract from each other. Although the topic of relative efficacy of combining treatment modalities is complex and beyond the scope of this chapter, it is also true that the effects of combined treatments are not invariably additive. In addition to uncertainty regarding the justification for combining medication and psychotherapy, there is little information to guide the optimal implementation of multimodal therapy. Therefore, current decisions regarding the sequencing and specific combinations of medication and psychotherapy treatments need to be based on individualized clinical and theoretical rationales.

Rationales for Medication Treatment Strategies: Evidence-Based Literature and Beyond

Clearly, the optimal basis for selecting a treatment option for PTSD or any other psychiatric disorder is demonstration of its efficacy in a randomized controlled trial. In this regard, the clinician can select an SSRI (particularly fluoxetine and sertraline) with confidence in many adult female patients with PTSD related to sexual and nonsexual assault. This is also the population in whom psychotherapeutic treatment has the best documented efficacy (Foa et al. 1999). The treatment literature on PTSD and general psychiatry can sometimes provide a basis for selecting medications for specific prominent symptom targets. For example, as previously noted, SSRIs benefit numbing symptoms (Brady et al. 2000; Conner et al. 1999; Tucker et al. 2001). Comorbidity within the spectrum of obsessive-compulsive disorder symptoms could also be uniquely responsive to these agents (Goodman et al. 1990). Findings from the depression literature (Armitage et al. 1997) and from open-label evaluations (Mellman et al. 1999) suggest that nefazodone and also trazodone (Ashford and Miller 1996) and guanfacine (an α-adrenergic blocker that is similar to clonidine) (Horrigan 1996) are

potentially beneficial for nightmares and sleep disturbance. Mood stabilizers have been suggested to successfully target volatility and impulsivity,
which are common target symptoms with PTSD, in other patient groups
(Stein et al. 1995).

In view of a bias for not publishing negative results, it seems that the
absence of evidence from randomized controlled trials of efficacy for SSRIs
in VA-based combat veterans warrants consideration. If one accepts that
this group is less responsive or nonresponsive to SSRIs, then it is potentially illuminating to explore why. Because the subjects of civilian PTSD
treatment studies are predominantly female, it is not possible at this time
to rule out a contribution of gender. Other considerations include factors
related to the type of trauma, chronicity and comorbidity, and effects of the
institutional disability system. It may also be worth noting that there were
earlier suggestions from open-label studies that SSRIs might have benefits
for veterans with combat-related PTSD (McDougle et al. 1991). This
author has been aware of apparent satisfaction with SSRI treatments
among patients diagnosed with PTSD and their prescribing clinicians in
the VA system. Thus, although SSRIs cannot be considered to be established treatments in male and veteran populations with PTSD, there may
be limitations of randomized controlled trials in reflecting benefits that
occur in nonresearch clinical populations. Limitations could be related to
measurement, recruitment, and/or other unidentified issues.

With regard to the treatment of combat veterans and of possible relevance to other male patient groups, the positive findings for tricyclic antidepressants and MAOIs are worth considering. A caveat to this
recommendation is the possibility that the veteran subjects recruited into
more recent studies may represent a group with more treatment-refractory
disease than the subjects of the studies conducted during the late 1980s on
tricyclic antidepressants and MAOIs. The available evidence-based literature is also limited or does not directly address cases in which comorbidity
is severe (i.e., primary) or is of a nature that would typically be a basis for
exclusion from a typical treatment study. Examples include concurrent sub-
stance-use disorders, psychotic symptoms, and histories of mania. For
these populations in particular, consideration of treatments with less extensive documentation as first-line therapies may be justified. Extrapolations
from the treatment literature for mood and other psychiatric disorders may
also be useful as a starting point for selecting and evaluating interventions.
Strategies for augmenting mood disorder treatment such as the addition of
lithium, other mood stabilizers, and new-generation antipsychotics (Nelson et al. 2000) warrant consideration for individual treatment and empirical evaluation of complex PTSD cases. Among the more commonly
extrapolated indications (e.g., anticonvulsants and novel antipsychotics for

impulsiveness and aggressivity within severe personality disorders [Chengappa et al. 1999; Stein et al. 1995]), it is worth noting that current documentation falls short of the standard of the randomized controlled trial.

As discussed in the beginning of the chapter, the development of treatments evolving more directly from knowledge of pathophysiology remains the goal for the field. Theoretical justification by no means obviates the need for empirical validation of treatment efficacy, however. Given the degree of speculation involved at present in treating PTSD, particularly the more complex cases, it is important that treatment effects be subject to ongoing critical evaluation. Interventions that have not clearly resulted in improvements should be discontinued and discontinuation effects, like treatment effects, should be carefully observed and ascertained. The clinician's utilization of some of the systematic rating tools referred to in Chapter 2 can be quite useful in this regard.

Integrating Medication Treatment With Psychotherapy

Because psychotherapy often has a principal role in the treatment of PTSD, another important consideration for using medication is its integration into a comprehensive treatment plan. As discussed in Chapter 3, specific psychotherapeutic approaches that involve direct exposure to the trauma memory have well-established efficacy for PTSD. As with medication, there are also open questions in the psychotherapy field regarding the extent of generalizability as well as tolerance of exposure techniques in more unstable subpopulations. As stated above, empirical studies do not directly address whether psychotherapy, medication, or their combination is advantageous in given situations. The often robust and enduring effects of specific psychotherapeutic techniques (see Chapter 3) justify their use as first-line therapies for many patients. Even when medication is a principal intervention and structured exposure or cognitive therapy is not being employed, the conduct of the therapeutic relationship is critical to achieving a successful outcome. Finally, although an advantage for combining medication and psychotherapy cannot be definitively asserted, the complex psychosocial and biological factors that contribute to the disorder would seem to justify such an approach in many cases.

One suggestion for integrating medication and psychotherapy in the treatment of PTSD is to establish an explicit rationale that can be discussed with the patient and, if applicable, the referring clinician. One rationale could be the lack of a complete response to initial treatment (e.g., an augmentation approach). Thus, medication might be prescribed when symptoms persist beyond a reasonable course of psychotherapy. There may also be scenarios in which medication and psychotherapy treatment might be considered to be potentially complementary or synergistic from the outset. This could include cases where comorbid conditions are prominent. Finally, medication might be considered the first-line intervention when symptoms are so severe that they would likely interfere with psychological processing.

There are a number of critical details that relate to how implementation of combined therapies is conducted. Sometimes a single clinician is responsible for both medication and psychological treatment. This situation may be optimal but it raises the challenge of a clinician being adequately apprised of developments in different modalities and not being unduly biased toward a particular technique or approach. Today it is common for treatments to be administered by clinicians with contrasting training and expertise. For combined treatment to be successful in these circumstances it is critical that the clinicians convey respect for each others' techniques, if they are reasonable. Relegating medication treatment to the status of an afterthought or an intervention of last resort could undermine a patient's confidence and likely compliance. Given the uncertainties regarding what constitute optimal treatments for the various presentations of PTSD, observing treatment response is often edifying for prescribing and referring clinicians as well as for the individual receiving the treatment.

References

American Psychiatric Association: Diagnostic and Statistical Manual of Mental Disorders, 3rd Edition. Washington, DC, American Psychiatric Association, 1980

American Psychiatric Association: Diagnostic and Statistical Manual of Mental Disorders, 4th Edition, Text Revision. Washington, DC, American Psychiatric Association, 2000

Armitage R, Yonkers K, Cole D, et al: A multicenter, double-blind comparison of the effects of nefazodone and fluoxetine on sleep architecture and quality of sleep in depressed outpatients. J Clin Psychopharmacol 17:161–168, 1997

Ashford JW, Miller TW: Effects of trazodone on sleep in patients diagnosed with post-traumatic stress disorder (PTSD). Journal of Contemporary Psychotherapy 26:221–233, 1996

Brady KT, Sonne SC, Roberts JM: Sertraline treatment of comorbid post-traumatic stress disorder and alcohol dependence. J Clin Psychiatry 56:502–505, 1995

Brady KT, Pearlstein T, Asnig GM, et al: Efficacy and safety of sertraline treatment of posttraumatic stress disorder: a randomized controlled trial. JAMA 283: 1837–1844, 2000

Braun P, Greenberg D, Dasberg H, et al: Core symptoms of post-traumatic stress disorder unimproved by alprazolam treatment. J Clin Psychiatry 51:236–238, 1990

Chengappa KNR, Ebeling T, Kang JS, et al: Clozapine reduces severe self-mutilation and aggression in psychotic patients with borderline personality disorder. J Clin Psychiatry 60:477–484, 1999

Conner KM, Southerland SM, Tuppler LA, et al: Fluoxetine in posttraumatic stress disorder. Br J Psychiatry 175:17–22,1999

Davidson JRT, Kudler H, Smith R, et al: Treatment of post-traumatic stress disorder with amitriptyline and placebo. Arch Gen Psychiatry 47:259–266, 1990

Fesler FA: Valproate in combat-related post-traumatic stress disorder. J Clin Psychiatry 52:361–364, 1991

Foa EB, Damar CV, Hambree EA, et al: The efficacy of exposure, stress inoculation, and their combination in ameliorating PTSD for female victims of assault. J Consult Clin Psychol 67:194–200, 1999

Frank JB, Kosten TR, Giller EL, et al: A randomized clinical trial of phenelzine and imipramine for post-traumatic stress disorder. Am J Psychiatry 1145:1289–1291, 1988

Friedman MJ, Southwick SM: Towards pharmacotherapy for PTSD, in Neurobiological and Clinical Consequences of Stress: From Normal Adaptation to PTSD. Edited by Friedman MJ, Charney DS, Deutch AY. Philadelphia, PA, Lippincott-Raven, 1995, pp 465–481

Goodman WK, Price LH, Delgado PL, et al: Specificity of serotonin reuptake inhibitors in the treatment of obsessive-compulsive disorder. Arch Gen Psychiatry 47:577–585, 1990

Hamner MB: Clozapine treatment for a veteran with comorbid psychosis and PTSD (letter). Am J Psychiatry 153:841, 1996

Hamner M, Ulmer H, Horne D: Buspirone potentiation of antidepressants in the treatment of PTSD. Depress Anxiety 5:137–139, 1997

Hidalgo R, Hertzberg MA, Mellman T: Nefazodone in post-traumatic stress disorder: results from six open-label trials. Int Clin Psychopharmacol 14(2):61–68, 1999

Hogben GL, Cornfeld RB: Treatment of traumatic war neurosis with phenelzine. Arch Gen Psychiatry 38:440–445, 1981

Horrigan JP: Guanfacine for PTSD nightmares. J Am Acad Child Adolesc Psychiatry 35:975–976, 1996

Kaplan Z, Amir M, Swartz M, et al: Inositol treatment of post-traumatic stress disorder. Anxiety 2:51–52, 1996

Kessler RC, Sonnega A, Bromet E, et al: Post-traumatic stress disorder in the National Comorbidity Survey. Arch Gen Psychiatry 52:1048–1060, 1995

Kolb LC, Burris BC, Griffiths S: Propranolol and clonidine in the treatment of post-traumatic stress disorders of war, in Post-Traumatic Stress Disorder: Psychological and Biological Sequelae. Edited by van der Kolk B. Washington, DC, American Psychiatric Press, 1984, pp 98–105

Lipper S, Davidson JRT, Grady TA, et al: Preliminary study of carbamazepine in post-traumatic stress disorder. Psychosomatics 27:849–854, 1986

Marmar CR, Schoenfeld F, Weiss CS, et al: Open trial of fluvoxamine for combat-related posttraumatic stress disorder. J Clin Psychiatry 57(suppl):66–72, 1996

Marshall RD, Schneier FR, Knight CBG, et al: An open trial of paroxetine in patients with noncombat-related chronic PTSD. J Clin Psychopharmacol 18:10–18, 1998

McDougle CJ, Southwick SM, Charney DS, et al: An open trial of fluoxetine in the treatment of posttraumatic stress disorder. J Clin Psychopharmacol 11:325–327, 1991

Mellman TA, David D, Barza L: Nefazodone treatment and dream reports in chronic PTSD. Depress Anxiety 9:146–148, 1999

Nagy LM, Southwick SM, Charney DS: Placebo-controlled trial of fluoxetine in PTSD. Poster presented at the International Society for Traumatic Stress Studies 12th Annual Meeting, San Francisco, CA, November 11, 1996

Nelson JC: Augmentation strategies in depression 2000. J Clin Psychiatry 61(suppl 2):13–19, 2000

Reist C, Kauffman CD, Haier RJ: A controlled trial of desipramine in 18 men with post-traumatic stress disorder. Am J Psychiatry 146:513–516, 1989

Shestatzky M, Greenberg D, Lerer B: A controlled trial of phenelzine in post-traumatic stress disorder. Psychiatry Res 24:149–155, 1988

Stein DJ, Simeon D, Frenkel M, et al: An open trial of valproate in borderline personality disorder. J Clin Psychiatry 56:506–510, 1995

Southwick SM, Krystal JH, Bremner JD, et al: Noradrenergic and serotonergic function in posttraumatic stress disorder. Arch Gen Psychiatry 54:749–758, 1997

Tucker P, Zannelli R, Yehuda R, et al: Paroxetine in the treatment of chronic post-traumatic stress disorder: results of a placebo-controlled, flexible-dosage trial. J Clin Psychiatry 62:860–868, 2001

van der Kolk BA, Dreyfull D, Michaels M, et al: Fluoxetine in post-traumatic stress disorder. J Clin Psychiatry 55:517–522, 1994

5

Treatment of Traumatized Children

Claude M. Chemtob, Ph.D.
Tisha L. Taylor, Psy.D.

Children are exposed to a wide range of traumatic life experiences. These can include physical and sexual abuse, war, displacement as refugees, natural and technical disasters, witnessing domestic violence, catastrophic illnesses, and motor vehicle accidents. Exposure to traumatic events can have wide-ranging behavioral and psychological consequences, including increased propensity to anger, aggression, suicidality, substance dependence, health care utilization, learning problems, and engaging in criminal acts (Giaconia et al. 1995). Psychiatric sequelae of childhood victimization also include developmental delays, increased anxiety and depressive symptoms, and sexually inappropriate and regressive behaviors (Kendall-Tackett et al. 1993). There is increasing recognition that childhood trauma can give rise to childhood posttraumatic stress disorder (PTSD).

Because trauma-related symptoms are associated with functional impairment and can adversely affect child development, traumatization of children and adolescents is a significant public health concern. Moreover, society incurs substantial direct and indirect costs as a result of child traumatization. For example, it has been estimated that each year more than 3 million children are maltreated (Poe-Yamagata 1997) and that direct services for these children currently cost over $20 billion annually (Peterson and Brown 1994). Beyond these direct costs, the impact of child victimization on families, schools, and communities is substantial. It results in parental lost workdays, social fragmentation, and lost potential.

Given that significant proportions of children exposed to traumatic events develop PTSD, there has been an increased interest in treating traumatic stress in children and adolescents. This chapter provides a review the efficacy of current treatments of child and adolescent PTSD and provides practical conceptual and technical guidelines for clinicians undertaking the treatment of traumatized children. Our goal is to increase sensitivity to developmental issues as they affect trauma treatment in general.

Childhood Victimization and PTSD

PTSD is the most frequently occurring disorder arising from exposure to traumatic events (Gurwitch et al. 1998). The symptoms of PTSD in children and adults are similar in many ways. However, in children reexperiencing symptoms may additionally include traumatic play involving the event and frightening dreams without recognizable content (in contrast to adults, who are more likely to have specific dreams of the event). As do adults, children with PTSD avoid reminders of the trauma and can develop attachment difficulties. Also, as do adults they frequently develop symptoms of hyperarousal and increased anger and aggression.

Prevalence of PTSD in Children

As in adult PTSD, estimates of the prevalence of PTSD in children show a wide range depending on factors relating to the type of event, timing, and nature of the assessment. However, unlike adult PTSD, there are no large scale epidemiological studies that have contributed population-based estimates of exposure to traumatic events and the resulting base rates of disorders (including PTSD) in children. According to the child literature, events involving the witnessing of parental murder, kidnapping, direct shooting or violence, and domestic violence are associated with the greatest prevalence of PTSD. Of children who witnessed a parental murder (Malmquist 1986), 100% were found to have PTSD. Terr (1981) reported 100% of children who had been involved in a school bus kidnapping showed posttraumatic emotional sequelae. Prevalence rates of PTSD have ranged from 27% of children exposed to a fatal school shooting (Schwarz and Kowalski 1991) to 60% of children exposed to a schoolground sniper attack (Pynoos et al. 1987). One year after a sniper attack, 74% of the children on the playground continued to show PTSD symptoms (Nader et al. 1990). Horowitz and colleagues (1995) reported that 67% of adolescent girls exposed to urban violence were diagnosed with PTSD. In a related context, Kinzie and colleagues (1986) reported that criteria for PTSD were met by 50% of adolescent Cambodian refugees. Of surviving siblings who lost a brother or sister due to an accidental death or homicide, 45% developed PTSD (Applebaum and Burns 1991). And of children exposed to domestic violence (Kilpatrick et al. 1997), 95% were found to have PTSD.

Researchers studying sexually abused children and physically abused children have found PTSD prevalence rates to vary across studies, yet the prevalence rates in cases of sexual abuse tend to be higher than in cases relating to physical abuse. In studies of sexually abused children, researchers (Deblinger et al. 1989; Dykman et al. 1997; Kiser et al. 1988; Livingston et al. 1993; McLeer et al. 1992, 1994) have reported PTSD prevalence rates ranging from 20.7% (Deblinger et al. 1989) to 90% (Kiser et al. 1988). Estimates of the prevalence of PTSD in physically abused children range from none (Pelcovitz et al. 1994) to 6.9% (Deblinger et al. 1989), to 23% (Dykman et al. 1997) and to 33% (Livingston et al. 1993). Studies of child physical and sexual abuse that have not differentiated the rates of PTSD associated with each type of abuse report prevalence ranging from 35% (Famularo et al.1994) to 39% (Famularo et al. 1992) to 50% (Dykman et al. 1997), and to 55% (Kiser et al. 1988). Combining rates appears to result in understating the effects of sexual abuse and inflating the effects of physical abuse.

Research has also examined PTSD as a sequela of life-threatening illnesses and automobile accidents and has found prevalence rates generally lower than those relating to violent and abusive situations. Pelcovitz and colleagues (1998) reported that 35% of adolescent subjects with cancer developed PTSD. Similarly, Stuber and colleagues (1991) reported that all the children they studied developed mild to moderate symptoms of PTSD after bone marrow transplants. Stallard and colleagues (1998) reported that 34.5% of children involved in a road traffic accident were found to have PTSD.

Children have also been found to develop PTSD after exposure to natural disasters; however, prevalence rates tend to be much lower than those described above, with the exception of a study involving children attending a school that experienced a high storm impact (Shaw et al. 1995). In a study that followed the Three Mile Island disaster, Handford and colleagues (1986) found no PTSD. Shannon and colleagues (1994) reported that after Hurricane Hugo, PTSD was found to range between 3.1% and 9.2%, depending on the child's age and sex. After Hurricane Andrew, which was a much more damaging hurricane, Garrison and colleagues (1995) found that 3% of adolescent boys and 9% of adolescent girls had PTSD, whereas LaGreca and colleagues (1996) reported 30% of children experiencing severe to very severe PTSD 3 months after Hurricane Andrew. Follow-up revealed 18% with severe or very severe PTSD at 7 months and 13% with severe or very severe PTSD after 10 months. In the study involving the high storm impact (which was also reporting on Hurricane Andrew), Shaw and colleagues (1995) reported exceptionally high PTSD prevalence of up to 87%. In 1991, Green and colleagues reported that of children exposed to the Buffalo Creek dam collapse, approximately 37% had a probable diagnosis of PTSD 2 years after the disaster. In considering the range of PTSD prevalence after natural disaster, it should be noted that natural disasters differ profoundly in their psychological impact. For example, the psychological characteristics of fears about radiation contamination resulting from a technological disaster such as the Three Mile Island nuclear power plant accident are quite different than the experience of direct exposure to a hurricane.

Efficacy of Current Treatments of Child and Adolescent PTSD

A review of the literature demonstrates that there are approximately 80 reports describing the treatment of childhood trauma; however, the majority of these papers are anecdotal. Only seven of the studies have examined the efficacy of one treatment compared with an alternative or no-treatment group. These studies are summarized in Table 5–1.

The studies were critically reviewed for adherence to rigorous standards of methodology. Foa and Meadows' (1997) "gold standards" for treatment outcome research (clearly defined target symptoms, reliable and valid measures, use of blind evaluators, assessor training, unbiased assignment to treatment, manualized treatment, and treatment adherence), as well as Kazdin and Weisz's (1998) and Kazdin's (1993, 1997) recommendations for evaluating empirically supported treatments guided this critical review. Table 5–2 outlines the adherence to these standards by the studies.

Of these seven studies, only two randomized, controlled studies directly evaluated the treatment of children with diagnosed PTSD. One focused on the treatment of sexually abused children (Deblinger et al. 1996), whereas the other focused on children with disaster-related PTSD (Chemtob et al., in press). A third study (March et al. 1998) addressed the treatment of children diagnosed with PTSD, but employed a "single-case-across-setting experimental design" (a quasi–waiting list design). This study only marginally met the comparison group design requirement. Although these three studies included a structured assessment of PTSD as a diagnosis by clinically trained assessors as part of their outcome measures, the remaining four studies assessed the impact of treatment on PTSD-

TABLE 5–1. Studies of traumatic stress with PTSD outcome measure

Study	Treatment and study type	Subjects	Treatment type/ length	Follow-up/ time since trauma	Past/ concurrent treatment	Findings
Deblinger et al. 1996	Individual CBT Controlled randomized	100, sexual abuse 25, child CBT 25, parent CBT 25, parent/ child CBT 25, community care 17 boys, 83 girls Mean age, 9.84 10 dropouts	12 weekly sessions: child or parent only (45 min); child/parent (90 min)	None/66% before 6 months, 16% 6 months to 2 years, 18% over 2 years	Not reported	Child and parent/child condition showed significant decreases in overall PTSD (K-SADS-E) compared with community care. Parent and parent/child conditions showed significant decreases in children's externalizing behavior (CBCL) and depression (CDI) and greater improvement in parenting skills (Parent Practices Questionnaire).
Chemtob et al. 2002	Individual EMDR Controlled randomized	32, natural disaster 17, EMDR 15, control 10 boys, 22 girls Mean age, 8.4 2 dropouts	EMDR treatment consisted of one diagnostic session and three weekly treatment sessions	6 months/3 years	Previous school-based brief psychosocial treatment	EMDR resulted in large reduction in level of symptoms on the Crisis Reaction Index, and significant reductions in anxiety (RCMAS) and depression (CDI). Treatment effects were maintained at 6-month follow-up.

TABLE 5–1. Studies of traumatic stress with PTSD outcome measure *(continued)*

Study	Treatment and study type	Subjects	Treatment type/ length	Follow-up/ time since trauma	Past/ concurrent treatment	Findings
March et al. 1998	Group CBT Single case across experimental setting	17, single-incident stressor 5 boys, 10 girls Mean age, 12.1 3 dropouts	18 group CBT sessions	6 months/ 1.5–2.5 years	None	57% no longer met criteria for PTSD (CATS; CAPS-C) at end of treatment, 86% no longer met criteria 6 months after treatment.
Chemtob et al., in press	Individual or group CBT vs. waiting list Controlled randomized	249, natural disaster 176, group CBT 73, individual CBT 97 boys, 152 girls Mean age, 8.2 34 dropouts	Four weekly individual or group CBT sessions with successive waves of 4–8 children serving as waiting list control subjects	1 year/2 years	Not reported	Posttreatment trauma symptoms (Kauai Reaction Index) significantly reduced with no difference between group and individual treatment.

TABLE 5–1. Studies of traumatic stress with PTSD outcome measure *(continued)*

Study	Treatment and study type	Subjects	Treatment type/ length	Follow-up/ time since trauma	Past/ concurrent treatment	Findings
Goenjian et al. 1997	Group and individual CBT Controlled comparison	63, natural disaster 35, CBT 29, control 22 boys, 41 girls Mean age, 13.2 No attrition	Four half-hour and two 1-hour trauma/grief-focused CBT brief therapy sessions over 3-week period	18 months after treatment/ 18 months after disaster	None	Experimental treatment resulted in alleviating PTSD (Child PTSD Reaction Index) symptoms and preventing worsening of depressive symptoms (Depression Self-Rating Scale) compared with the control group.
Celano et al. 1996	Individual CBT plus metaphoric techniques Controlled randomized	47, sexual abuse 15, CBT 17, supportive therapy 32 girls and mothers Mean age, 10.5 15 dropouts	1-hour sessions for 8 weeks, half session with mother and half with child	None/within 1 to 26 months after abuse	None had received treatment for abuse	Both groups showed decreased PTSD (CITIES-R) and internalizing and externalizing behavior (CBCL). No change noted in betrayal and sex-related beliefs. CBT showed decrease in caretaker self-blame and expectations of undue negative impact on the child.

TABLE 5–1. Studies of traumatic stress with PTSD outcome measure *(continued)*

Study	Treatment and study type	Subjects	Treatment type/ length	Follow-up/ time since trauma	Past/ concurrent treatment	Findings
Yule 1992	Group CBT Controlled comparison	39, accident 24, CBT 15, control 39 girls Age, 4–15 years No attrition	Debriefing meeting 10 days after the disaster. Two small open groups	None/5 to 9 months	Not reported	After 5–9 months, treatment group showed significantly lower scores on the Impact of Events Scale and on fear survey.

Note. CAPS-C=Clinician-Administered PTSD Scale–Child and Adolescent Version; CATS=Child Abuse and Trauma Scale; CBCL=Child Behavior Checklist; CBT=cognitive–behavioral therapy; CDI=Child Depression Inventory; CITIES-R=Children's Impact of Traumatic Events Scales–Revised; EMDR=eye movement desensitization and reprocessing; K-SADS-E=Schedule for Affective Disorders and Schizophrenia for School-Age Children; RCMAS=Revised Children's Manifest Anxiety Scale.

TABLE 5–2. Gold standards for treatment outcome: studies with traumatic stress outcome measures

Study	PTSD or trauma symptoms	Clearly defined target symptoms	Reliable valid measures	Blind evaluators	Assessor training	Manualized replicable specific treatment	Random assignment	Treatment adherence
Deblinger et al. 1996	PTSD	Yes	Yes	No	Yes	Yes	Yes	Yes
Chemtob al. 2002	PTSD	Yes	Yes	Yes	Yes	Yes	Yes	Yes
March et al. 1998	PTSD	Yes	Yes	No	Not reported	Yes	No	Not reported
Chemtob al., in press	Trauma symptoms	Yes	Yes	Yes	Yes	Yes	Yes	Supervision only
Goenjian et al. 1997	Trauma symptoms	Yes	Yes	Not reported	Yes	Not reported	No	Not reported
Celano et al. 1996	Trauma symptoms	Yes	Yes	Yes	Yes	Yes	Yes	Supervision only
Yule 1992	Trauma symptoms	Yes	Yes	No	Not reported	No	No	Not reported

related trauma symptoms, primarily using self-report measures.

In the first of the three studies, Deblinger and colleagues (1996) reported on a controlled randomized treatment study aimed at determining the efficacy of short-term cognitive-behavioral treatment with sexually abused school-age children experiencing PTSD symptoms. The design compared three treatment conditions (a child-only intervention, a parent-only intervention, and combined child and parent intervention) to standard therapeutic care received in the community.

Participants included 100 sexually abused children recruited from community sources. Children ranged in age from 7 to 13, with a mean age of 9.84. Eighty-three percent of the participants were girls, including 72% Caucasian, 20% African-American, 6% Hispanic, and 2% other. The majority of the participating children had experienced the abuse within the past 6 months, whereas the rest had been abused during the previous 6-month to 2-year period. The children were clinically assessed and the group was found to be characterized by the following diagnoses: 71%, PTSD; 29%, major depression; 30%, oppositional defiant disorder; 20%, attention-deficit disorder; 11%, separation anxiety; 10%, overanxious; 6%, conduct disorder; 5%, specific phobia; and 1%, obsessive-compulsive disorder. Clearly, a large number of the children had substantial psychopathology.

Subjects were randomly assigned to conditions. No significant differences were found between the subjects in the four treatment conditions based on sex, age, ethnicity, identity of the perpetrator, frequency of contact sexual abuse, type of contact sexual abuse, use of force, and the pretreatment conditions. No significant differences were found between the 10 subjects who did not return for the posttreatment assessment compared with those who did complete treatment, except that the 10 subjects who did not return experienced significantly fewer incidents of contact sexual abuse.

The child intervention was described as consisting of a number of cognitive-behavioral methods, including gradual exposure, modeling, education, coping, and body safety skills training. The parent intervention combined several cognitive-behavioral strategies and involved application of these strategies in direct work with the child. Thus, the therapist taught the parents skills for responding therapeutically to their children's behaviors and needs through the use of modeling, gradual exposure, and supporting cognitive processing. Both interventions comprised 12 sessions. Participants in the community control condition were provided information about their children's symptoms and were strongly encouraged to seek therapy.

Therapists in the experimental treatment conditions were described as mental health therapists and were required to follow a detailed treatment manual. They received intensive didactic training in the experimental treatment approach and used the treatment in one pilot case. Therapists also completed therapy procedure checklists for each session and participated in intensive weekly supervision, frequently using their audiotape sessions.

Target symptoms for treatment were defined as children's behavior problems, anxiety, depression, PTSD symptoms, and parenting practices. Instruments used to assess the children were the State-Trait Anxiety Inventory for Children (Spielberger 1973), Child Depression Inventory (M. Kovacs, "The Child Depression Inventory: A Self-Rated Depression Scale for School-Aged Youngsters," unpublished manuscript, University of Pittsburgh School of Medicine, 1983), Child Behavior Checklist (Achenbach and Edelbrock 1991), and Parenting Practices Questionnaire (Knight et al. 1982). The PTSD section of the Schedule for Affective Disorders and Schizophrenia for School-Age Children (K-SADS-E) (Chambers et al. 1985) was used to diagnose PTSD. The therapist and a clinical research assistant collected the baseline assessment data over the course of two assessment periods. In addition, the therapist conducted the structured background and the K-SADS-E diagnostic interview (except the PTSD section), whereas the clinical research assistant administered all outcome measures including the PTSD section of the K-SADS-E and the parent and child self-report measures.

After treatment, PTSD symptoms (as assessed by K-SADS-E) were reduced when the child was included in treatment (the child-only and parent-child conditions). When a parent was included in treatment (parent-only and parent-child conditions), there were significantly greater decreases in children's externalizing behaviors (assessed by the Child Behavior Checklist) and depression (assessed by the Children's Depression Inventory) and more improvement in parenting skills (assessed by the Parenting Practices Questionnaire). Of the 25 children in the community control condition, 12 received treatment in the community. These children were compared with the 13 community control children who did not receive treatment. No difference was found between the two groups on the seven outcome scores.

The study design was notable for its inclusion of measures of PTSD symptoms as well as measures of depression, anxiety, and externalizing behavior. This provided an expanded perspective on the impact of the treatment. Information on the number and background of the therapists providing treatment and evaluating changes in comorbid psychopathology was not reported. Although impressive plans for extended follow-up at 3, 6, 12, and 24 months were described, the lack of follow-up information and the failure to use assessors blind to treatment condition limit confidence in the results of this otherwise ambitious study.

The second study (Chemtob et al. 2002) was a randomized, controlled school-based treatment study using eye movement desensitization and reprocessing (EMDR). Participants were 32 children from seven different schools on Kauai who met criteria for PTSD 3 years after exposure to Hurricane Iniki, as well as 1 year after a brief school-based, counselor-administered psychosocial treatment. The study included children in grades 2–6 with a mean age of 8.4 years. There were 22 girls and 10 boys with 28% Filipino, 31% Hawaiian (or part), 12.5% Japanese, 19% Caucasian, and 9.5% mixed ethnic origins. In comparing the immediate and delayed treatment groups, no differences were found on gender, grade, socioeconomic level (as measured by free lunch status), age, exposure, or Kauai Recovery Index (KRI) (Hamada et al. 1996) scores.

The authors described EMDR as a client-paced exposure treatment that incorporates elements of psychodynamic treatments. The protocol provided for one diagnostic session and three weekly treatment sessions; in addition a written step-by-step treatment protocol was followed. Four doctoral-level clinicians (three men and one woman) provided the EMDR therapy. All were experienced clinicians who had completed at least Level I EMDR training. An experienced EMDR child clinical psychologist conducted 16 hours of child EMDR training. All treatment sessions were videotaped. To ensure adherence to EMDR, each therapist reviewed five of each other's videotaped sessions on a rotating basis. Furthermore, the therapists received frequent feedback from one of the researchers, and therapists met weekly as a group for 4 hours to review each other's treatment tapes.

Target symptoms were PTSD symptoms, clinically evaluated using the Children's Reaction Inventory (CRI) (Pynoos et al. 1987), and associated symptoms as measured by the Revised Children's Manifest Anxiety Scale (Reynolds and Richmond 1985) and the Child Depression Inventory. The KRI was used to screen children for the study. Visits to the school health nurse and Child Ratings of Treatment Helpfulness provided additional information. Independent examiners blind to group assignment administered the psychometric assessment instruments. The children's therapists administered the CRI to guide their clinical assessment of PTSD. The diagnostic interviews were videotaped and reviewed by a second clinician to offset possible interviewer bias. To be included in the study, a participant had to be identified as having PTSD by both evaluators.

Both groups showed large reductions in PTSD symptoms as measured by the CRI. They also showed significant reductions in both anxiety (assessed by the Revised Children's Manifest Anxiety Scale), and depression (assessed by the Children's Depression Inventory). These gains were maintained at 6 months. An additional finding was a reduction in the visits to the school nurse by children in the remitted group. Clinical significance was addressed by evaluating the number of children who no longer met criteria for PTSD and by identifying at both pretreatment and follow-up assessments the number of children in each severity category on the CRI. Results showed a reduction in the number of children in the moderate and severe categories and an increase in the number of children scoring in the mild category.

The finding of the effectiveness of EMDR with a multicultural population of children is an important addition to the treatment literature, and the results are impressive, especially given the brevity of treatment. Clinical significance was addressed through a 6-month follow-up, which showed that changes were maintained or improved. The finding of reductions in the number of visits to the school nurse among the remitted children buttressed the phenomenological findings of improved symptom outcomes.

Evaluation of possible comorbid diagnoses would have been useful, given the fact that not all of the children improved. It is possible that the children who did not improve had additional trauma or other psychopathology. The study design did not evaluate the impact of the passage of time on PTSD symptoms among children in the waiting-list condition. However, there was no change due to the passage of time on self-report measures of depression or anxiety, and the children in the study were identified on the basis of the persistence of their symptoms 3 years after the disaster and lack of response to prior treatment. The findings of this study are limited because it did not provide for independent assessors or an active comparison treatment.

In the third study, March and colleagues (1998) used a single case-across-setting experimental design (a quasi-experimental waiting list control group design) to validate a new treatment described as multimodality trauma treatment. The impact of the treatment on symptoms of PTSD—as well as on anxiety, anger, depression, and externalizing behaviors in children and adolescents—was evaluated. Participants were recruited through screening for PTSD all children in grades 4–9 at two elementary and two junior high schools ($N=1,800$) in a small southeastern town. Treatment participants were 17 children and adolescents with a diagnosis of PTSD, ranging in age from 10 to 15 years with a mean age of 12.1. The authors reported that the participants were 10 girls and 5 boys (inconsistent with their report of 17 total participants), with 7 of them being black, 1 Asian, 1 American Indian, and 8 white. Ten participants had experienced two or more traumatic events, whereas 7 experienced a single trauma. The average duration of PTSD symptoms was 1.5 years for elementary school children and 2.5 years for adolescents. Stressors experienced by the subjects were automobile accidents, severe storms, accidental injury, severe illness, accidental and criminal gunshot injury, and fires. Stressors that happened to a loved one included death by criminal assault, illness, automobile accidents, death by fire, and gunshot injury.

The manual-driven multimodality trauma treatment protocol, an 18-week group cognitive-behavioral treatment, was based on social learning theory coupled with a current understanding of the social and biological bases of PTSD. Each session included a statement of goals, careful review of the previous week's work, introduction of new information, therapist-assisted "nuts and bolts" practice, homework for the coming week, and monitoring procedures. Treatment sessions included getting started, naming and mapping, anxiety management training 1 and 2, grading feelings, anger coping 1 and 2, cognitive training 1 and 2, introducing exposure and response prevention, pullout session, trial exposure, narrative exposure 1 and 2, worst moment exposure 1 and 2, right beliefs, relapse prevention, generalization, and a graduation party. No information was provided about the individuals who led the treatment groups.

The target symptoms were clearly defined. They included PTSD symptoms as measured by the Clinician-Administered PTSD Scale–Child and Adolescent Version (Nader et al. 1994), the Clinical Global Improvement Scale (Endicott et al. 1976), the Conners Teachers Rating Scale for externalizing symptoms (Conners 1969), the Multidimensional Anxiety Scale for Children (March et al. 1977), the Children's Depression Inventory, and the trait subscale of the State-Trait Anger Expression Inventory (Spielberger et al. 1985). The Nowicki-Strickland "What I Am Like" scale (Norwicki and Strickland 1973) was used to index locus of control. Blind evaluators were not used.

Fifty-seven percent of the subjects completing treatment no longer met diagnostic criteria for PTSD at posttreatment assessment. At the 6-month follow-up, 86% of the participants were free of PTSD symptoms. All other outcome measures except the Conners Teachers Rating Scale (which was within normal range at pretreatment assessment) showed marked improvement at posttreatment assessment and 6-month follow-up. The locus of control measure displayed no treatment effect between pretreatment and posttreatment assessments; however, a robust change in the direction of internal locus of control was shown between posttreatment and follow-up assessments.

The success of the use of a group approach with children who had experienced different types of trauma is a significant finding indicating the usefulness of a single model of intervention for different traumatized populations. The authors used a manualized treatment protocol, assessed for PTSD and other pathology associated with PTSD, and provided treatment for a variety of stressors that caused PTSD. In addition, the screening approach had merit and may prove to be useful in other types of trauma-detection situations. The use of intent-to-treat analytical methods that account for missing data represented a step forward in the analysis of data in this field.

Unfortunately, there were some methodological problems that limit the generalizability of the findings of this study. Although the authors asserted that the single case across time, across location, and across school type (age) controlled for factors such as passage of time and maturation, a comparison treatment control group was absent. Thus, the study did not account for the general effects of therapeutic attention that may have been the reason for improvement. Also, the children were tested every other week, which may have created demand characteristics due to the constant testing. It is possible that a no-treatment control group that was tested every other week with the same instruments may have also shown improvement. Furthermore, participants were highly screened; to be included in treatment, children had to have high motivation to work on PTSD symptoms, cognitive ability, and social problem-solving skills. Subjects who experienced abuse-related PTSD and those with conduct problems were excluded. This appears to limit generalizability to smarter, better adjusted, and socially capable individuals. Blind evaluators were not used, and subjects were not randomized to groups. Information on treatment integrity was also incomplete.

In the most recent of the four studies assessing the impact of treatment on PTSD-related trauma symptoms, Chemtob and colleagues (in press) conducted a school-based randomized, controlled study with elementary school children 2 years after Hurricane Iniki. The goal of this study was to determine the feasibility of identifying children with persistent traumatic stress symptoms 2 years after the disaster, as well as to assess the efficacy of providing psychosocial treatment to affected children. A secondary goal was to compare group treatment and individual treatment. All children in Kauai's 10 public elementary schools attending 2nd through 6th grades ($N=4,258$) were screened. Children reporting the most severe trauma symptoms were assigned to treatment (approximately 5% of the screened population). Of the 249 children meeting the screening criteria, 215 completed treatment (86.3%). Of these 215, 61.4% were girls and 38.6% were boys, ranging in age from 6 to 12 with a mean age of 8.2 years. The ethnic breakdown of the subjects was 30.1% Hawaiian or part Hawaiian, 24.9% Caucasian, 19.7% Filipino, and 9.2% Japanese. Because of limitations in treatment capacity, the investigators randomized children into three treatment waves. There was approximately a 1-month lag from the end of treatment for one group until the beginning of treatment for the next group.

The second and third groups served as waiting list control subjects.

The intervention philosophy assumed that most children recover naturally from a disaster by mastering disaster-related psychological challenges. Children who do not recover are presumed to have been unable to master one or more of these psychological challenges. The authors described their intervention as being designed to restart and support completion of these psychological challenges. They proposed that such challenges for the child are 1) to successfully restore a sense of safety, 2) to adaptively grieve losses and renew attachments, 3) to express and resolve disaster-related anger, and 4) to achieve closure about the disaster to move forward.

Separate protocols were written for the individual and the group treatment. Treatment was manual-guided and developmentally appropriate. Three days of training regarding postdisaster trauma psychology and 12 hours of didactic training specific to the treatment manual were provided. Four therapists—two women and two men—three of whom were school counselors and one a clinical social worker, provided therapy. Three hours of group supervision was provided weekly, for 4 weeks, in the course of which the therapists presented their work orally and received supervision aimed at maximizing treatment uniformity. Each group included four to eight children.

Outcome measures included the 24-item self-report KRI, which measured the self-reported frequency of symptoms keyed to DSM-IV (American Psychiatric Association 1994), and the clinician-administered CRI. The person administering the pretreatment and posttreatment outcome measures (the KRI) was the child's therapist. As a converging measure of outcome, the CRI was administered to a randomly drawn subset of treated and untreated children ($N=44$) by clinicians blind to whether the child had been provided treatment. Results on both the KRI and the CRI showed that treated children had fewer symptoms than untreated children. Posttreatment scores showed significant reductions on the KRI. There were no differences between those who received group treatment and those who received individual treatment. At 1-year follow-up assessment, treated children showed no resurgence of trauma-related symptoms.

This field study was the first randomized, controlled study to evaluate the treatment of trauma symptoms in a postdisaster context. Two important findings were reported. First is the finding that brief psychosocial intervention was efficacious for most of the treated children, and second is that group intervention was as effective as individual treatment. There are several weaknesses in this study, which limit generalization of the findings. The authors did not assess possible comorbid diagnoses, which allows for the possibility that the children who did not improve had other psychopathology complicating their PTSD. Attrition was only partially addressed, as the authors did not report whether the dropouts had significantly different scores on any of the assessment instruments. The same therapists who conducted the therapy administered the KRI, which may have created demand characteristics. Also, video/audio taping the sessions with review by an independent assessor for treatment fidelity would have strengthened the findings.

Goenjian and colleagues (1997) evaluated the effectiveness of a school-based intervention by comparing scores for PTSD and depressive symptoms before and after intervention among treated and untreated groups in an Armenian city devastated by an earthquake. Participants included 64 early adolescents from four schools. Students at two of the schools participated in trauma/grief-focused brief psychotherapy ($N=35$), whereas students at the other two schools were not treated ($N=29$). Three years after the earthquake, the mean age of the subjects was 13.2 years. The only statistical comparison of the two groups was by age and numbers of males and females. The treated group included 11 boys and 24 girls with a mean age of 13.2, compared with 11 boys and 18 girls with a mean age of 13.3 in the untreated group.

Due to the limited number of mental health personnel, the two schools closest to the authors' clinic were chosen for treatment. The damage to the four schools and their neighborhoods were the same, and there were no socioeconomic differences between the groups. There was no attrition; in addition, none of the students had received mental health treatment beyond this intervention, had a history of substance abuse, or were prescribed psychotropic medication during the study. The subjects participated in four half-hour group sessions and two to four 1-hour individual sessions over a 3-week period. The treatment sessions were completed during a 6-week period approximately 1.5 years after the earthquake. The trauma/grief-focused treatment addressed five major areas: 1) trauma reconstruction and reprocessing, 2) trauma reminders, 3) postdisaster stresses and adversities, 4) bereavement and the interplay of trauma and grief, and 5) developmental impact. Drawings, discussions, problem solving, relaxation, and reframing techniques were used. No information was reported about the therapists providing treatment.

The target symptoms were defined as PTSD symptomatology and depressive reactions. Outcome measures included the Child Posttraumatic Stress Disorder Reaction Index (Nader et al. 1990) and the Depression Self-Rating Scale (Asarnow and Carlson 1985). Trained mental health professionals administered the assessment instruments. There was no mention of whether the evaluators were blind to treatment condition.

Results showed that the experimental group had reduced posttraumatic stress symptoms, and there were no changes in depressive symptoms compared with the no-treatment control group. Even though PTSD symptoms were reduced, they remained in the clinical range for the treated group. In the no-treatment control group, both posttraumatic stress and depressive symptoms increased.

Given the limitations inherent in research targeting a disaster of this magnitude, the study was well conducted. Strengths included use of individual and group modalities, follow-up 18 months after treatment, and clearly defined target symptoms. The study supports the value of providing even brief intervention to support the recovery of traumatized students after a natural disaster. This investigation would have been improved by using random assignment to groups and a manualized treatment protocol, by providing a statistical comparison of the two groups on demographic variables, and by including measures of treatment adherence.

Celano and colleagues (1996) used a pre-post randomized experimental design to compare the efficacy of two short-term treatment programs for sexually abused girls and their nonoffending female caretakers. The experimental treatment was based on Finkelhor and Browne's (1985) theoretical model (known as "RAP" [Responding to Abuse Program] treatment, described below) and "treatment as usual," defined as the supportive, unstructured psychotherapy that sexually abused girls and their mothers would ordinarily receive at the clinic.

Subjects were recruited from the pediatric emergency clinic of a large public hospital (66%), the local statutory child protection agencies (28%), and victims' assistance programs of the court system (7%). Participants included 32 girls and their nonoffending female caretakers. The girls ranged in age from 8 to 13 with a mean age of 10.5. The sample consisted primarily of African-American families (75%), as well as Caucasian (22%) and Hispanic (3%) families. Female caretakers ranged in age from 24 to 61 (mean age, 36). There was no significant difference between the two treatment groups in the length of the interval between disclosure and treatment, and none of the subjects had received treatment for the abuse before their participation in the study. There were no significant differences between subjects in the RAP and treatment as usual interventions relative to child's age or race, relationship of perpetrator, abuse severity, caretaker's history of child sexual abuse, relationship of caretaker to the child, and therapist experience. Fifteen families dropped out after treatment began. The relative percentage of families that dropped out did not differ between the two treatment groups. There were also no differences for the child's age or race, relationship of the perpetrator, abuse severity, caretaker's abuse history, relationship of caretaker to child, and pretreatment scores on the dependent measures.

The RAP program consisted of eight sessions, with approximately two sessions addressing each dimension of Finkelhor's four-factor model. The first two sessions included activities designed to address blame and stigmatization. Sessions 3 and 4 addressed children's feelings of betrayal related to their victimization, and sessions 5 and 6 addressed traumatic sexualization, that is, the process by which a child victim's sexual attitudes, feelings, and behaviors are shaped in a developmentally inappropriate and interpersonally dysfunctional manner as a result of the abuse. The last two sessions were devoted to the issue of powerlessness and concomitant anxiety in an effort to decrease the child's abuse-related anxiety and helplessness and improve assertiveness skills. The parent intervention component targeted self-blame and stigmatization, sense of betrayal by the perpetrator, understanding and coping with manifestations of impact on the child's sexuality of the trauma, and perceptions of powerlessness.

The program was theoretically based and devoted equal time to non-offending parents and child victims. In addition, the treatment was designed to be culturally sensitive to the needs of a primarily low-income, African-American sample, an underserved and understudied population. The therapeutic materials included a rap song and utilized illustrations of African-American children. This treatment program used developmentally appropriate cognitive-behavioral and metaphoric techniques to address children's maladaptive beliefs, affect, and behavior along these four dimensions. A treatment manual outlined the theoretical rationale and specific treatment activities of the RAP.

The therapists were 18 women psychiatrists, psychologists, social workers, nurses, and trainees in psychiatry and psychology with prior education and experience in psychotherapy with children. All therapists were provided with additional training and supervision in the area of child sexual abuse. Therapists providing the experimental treatment participated in a 3-hour training session before beginning treatment as well as weekly supervision in the use of the RAP curriculum. Trainees providing treatment as usual received weekly supervision highlighting clinical issues relevant to child sexual abuse. Professional clinicians utilizing treatment as usual participated in monthly group supervision sessions.

Target symptoms were defined as psychosocial functioning, traumatogenic beliefs, self-blame, and powerlessness. A structured interview developed by the project investigators was used to obtain information from the caretaker about demographic data, the child's history of abuse and current psychosocial functioning, the caretaker's history of child sexual abuse (if any), past psychiatric history of caretaker and child, and perceptions of disruption to the family as a result of the abuse disclosure. Child outcome measures included the Child Behavior Checklist (Achenbach 1991) and the

Children's Global Assessment Scale (Shaffer et al. 1983) to measure a child's psychosocial functioning and PTSD and Children's Impact of Traumatic Events Scales–Revised (Wolfe et al. 1991) to measure PTSD, self-blame, betrayal, traumatic sexualization, and powerlessness. Maternal outcome measures included the Parental Attribution Scale (Everson et al. 1989) and Parent Reaction to Incest Disclosure Scale (Everson et al. 1989) to measure self-blame, child blame, perpetrator blame, and negative impact. A clinician blind to treatment condition completed the assessments both before and after treatment.

Results indicated that subjects in both the structured RAP treatment and the relatively unstructured treatment as usual intervention improved very similarly on almost all treatment measures. Children in both groups reported a decrease in beliefs reflecting self-blame and powerlessness. Neither group changed in betrayal-related beliefs or sex-related beliefs. The RAP treatment was more effective than treatment as usual in increasing abuse-related caretaker support of the child and decreasing self-blame and expectations of undue negative impact of the abuse on the child. No changes in Parental Attribution Scale scores of child blame or perpetrator blame were found for either group. Clinicians reported that the structured RAP activities were helpful to them in organizing their conceptual and clinical work, which may be particularly advantageous for less experienced clinicians.

This was a theoretically based, methodologically sound and culturally sensitive study in which the theoretical basis defined the target symptoms. The sample description was thorough, the groups were randomly assigned relative to RAP and treatment as usual, and dropouts showed no statistical differences. In addition, the study targeted specific symptoms with valid measures and included a detailed treatment manual. Inclusion and exclusion criteria were well defined, and the authors provided a thorough sample description and discussed past and concurrent treatment. However, the study did not discuss comorbid diagnoses or the clinical significance of findings and did not include any follow-up data. Video/audio taping treatment sessions to ensure adherence to the treatment objectives would have improved treatment integrity. The dropout rate was quite high, as 34% of the families did not complete treatment.

The last of the four studies, by Yule (1992), compared the effects of a school-based early intervention after a ship accident at two girls' schools, where one school accepted an offer of outside help and the other did not. The subjects were 39 girls who survived a ship accident while on a school outing. There were 24 girls in the experimental group and 15 in the control group. No other demographic information was provided. A debriefing meeting was held 10 days after the disaster for all survivors. Two small open groups met and were based on a problem-solving approach using cognitive-behavioral methods to target symptoms of anxiety, avoidance, and intrusive thoughts. The intervention did not include a manual, and information was not included for replication. There was no information on treatment adherence. Outcome measures included the Fear Survey Schedule for Children (Ollendick et al. 1991), Revised Children's Manifest Anxiety Scale (Reynolds and Richmond 1978), Birleson Depression Inventory (Birleson 1981), and Horowitz's Revised Impact of Events Scale (Horowitz et al. 1979). There was no information on who administered the assessment instruments.

Results indicated that, 5–9 months later, the school in the experimental group showed significantly lower scores on the Impact of Events Scale, with a stronger showing on intrusion than on avoidance items. The anxiety and depression scores were slightly, but not significantly, lower. The experimental group reported significantly fewer fears overall, with treatment effect being stronger for fears unrelated to the accident than those related to the accident on the Fear Survey Schedule.

The study barely met the criteria for inclusion in this review. The author did not provide crucial information for critical evaluation. There was no description of inclusion and exclusion criteria, sample characteristics, differences between the experimental and control groups, past and concurrent treatment, or comorbid diagnoses. There was an incomplete description of the treatment, and it was not manualized for future replication.

Although this early postdisaster treatment study supports the value of offering treatment to traumatized children, its findings are severely limited by the use of two groups that may have differed on a large number of variables. It is difficult to ascertain that the improvement among the treated adolescents is attributable to the effects of treatment. Differential selection, as well as differences in the school environment after the event and after treatment, could potentially account for the different symptomatic outcomes.

Current Status of Empirical Literature

The purpose of this section is to evaluate whether efficacious treatment for traumatized children and adolescents experiencing PTSD symptoms is currently available. The first issue addressed is whether treatment is more effective than no treatment in reducing trauma symptoms. Five of the seven studies reviewed (Chemtob et al. 2002, in press; Goenjian et al. 1997; March et al. 1998; Yule 1992) compared an experimental treatment condition to a waiting list or no-treatment control group. Each of these studies found the treatment condition to be more effective than the control group. In all of the studies, the period of time since the trauma exceeded 3 months, which suggests that symptoms persisted for at least 3 months without spontaneous remission and were not ameliorating merely due to the passage of time. On the other hand, improvement relative to no treatment is consistent with Kazdin's (1997) view that changes associated with treatment generally are greater than those found in groups not receiving formal treatment. Therefore, the findings of most of the studies reviewed cannot rule out that the treatment effects merely reflected increased attention to the children's needs.

Two of the studies provided controls for the general effects of therapeutic attention and permitted further examination of this issue. Deblinger et al. (1996) and Celano et al. (1996) compared different treatments, each presumed to be active, rather than merely using waiting list no-treatment control groups. Deblinger et al. (1996) found differences between their several treatment conditions, which suggest treatment-specific effects. Specifically, both the child treatment conditions resulted in reductions in the child-centered measures of symptoms, whereas in both the parent treatment conditions the parent-centered measures reflected treatment-related improvements. The combined parent-child treatment condition was more effective than the other conditions. The authors interpreted these findings as reflecting specific effects of treatment. However, the alternative interpretation is that the parent-child treatment was more effective in reducing symptoms because participants received twice as much treatment. It is also problematic that of the children who were randomly assigned to the community care control group, those who received community-based routine treatment did not differ in outcome from the members of the control group who did not receive such care. This suggests that the community treatment comparison was not an active treatment. Regrettably, the key comparison required to address this issue, namely whether the children who had received community care differed from the children who received the experimental treatment, was not reported. Without evaluating such comparisons, it is impossible to conclusively rule out the general effects of therapeutic attention. Further adding to the need for caution in interpreting the findings of Deblinger and colleagues, Celano et al. (1996) found that both cognitive-behavioral treatment and supportive counseling were equally effective in reducing trauma symptoms.

Remarkably, only three studies focused directly on the treatment of PTSD. These studies used PTSD as inclusion criteria, whereas the remaining four studies measured PTSD-related trauma symptoms as targets for treatment. Deblinger et al. (1996) used an individual CBT protocol, whereas March et al. (1998) used a group CBT protocol. Chemtob and colleagues used EMDR, an individual treatment. All three research groups reported reductions in PTSD rates as a function of treatment. Unfortunately, March and colleagues used a quasi–waiting-list experimental method, did not randomly assign participants to treatment conditions, and did not report on the effectiveness of their therapeutic fidelity controls. Chemtob et al. (in press) used a no-treatment control group, whereas Deblinger and colleagues failed to use blind evaluators. Even given these limitations, all three studies reported substantial reduction in PTSD symptoms in children with chronic PTSD. These data support cautious optimism with respect to the treatment of PTSD in children and adolescents.

Variants of cognitive-behavioral therapy (CBT) were used in six (Celano et al. 1996; Chemtob et al. 1999; Deblinger et al. 1996; Goenjian et al. 1997; March et al. 1998; Yule 1992) of the seven studies in this review. Four of the studies used either a no-treatment or a waiting-list control group, so the comparison was between treatment and no treatment, and two studies compared active treatment conditions (Celano et al. 1996; Deblinger et al. 1996). The results of these studies, with the exception of the study by Celano and colleagues, showed CBT to be more efficacious than control conditions. The study by Celano and colleagues showed no difference between individual CBT and supportive counseling. The results of the study by Deblinger and colleagues suggested that CBT might be more effective than routine community care (see the discussion above). These latter two studies are more informative because they included a control for the general effects of therapeutic attention (and other nonspecific treatment effects such as therapist and rater expectations), and their results make it impossible to say whether CBT is more effective than other kinds of treatment.

Moreover, it should be noted that the six CBT studies described different treatment packages. Despite a common label, the actual treatment procedures differed widely. Deblinger and colleagues (1996) and March and colleagues (1998) specifically reported using exposure, in addition to a variety of other CBT techniques. Unfortunately, it is not possible from the existing studies to determine whether exposure treatment specifically contributed to the success of these treatments. This is a common problem because outcome studies frequently report beneficial effects but rarely identify "effective" ingredients (Kazdin and Weisz 1998).

One non-CBT study also showed efficacy. A study by Chemtob and colleagues (2002) used EMDR as a treatment for PTSD symptoms. Their results showed a large reduction in symptoms and large effect sizes. Although the authors noted that symptoms had not remitted despite prior treatment, confidence in the findings would have been greater if another clinical treatment (in addition to a waiting list control group) had been used. What is known at this time is that EMDR treatment led to reduced symptoms, but as with CBT, it cannot be excluded that this was due to non-specific effects of treatment. Because EMDR is a streamlined and cost-effective treatment, replication with other traumatized populations and the use of an active treatment comparison would provide valuable information on the efficacy of this treatment.

The studies reviewed converge to suggest that structured treatment focusing on PTSD and trauma symptoms can substantially ameliorate the effects of child and adolescent trauma. Unfortunately, current treatment providers generally tend to use counseling approaches. These are usually found to be less effective (Fonagy 1997).

Child and adolescent PTSD treatment efficacy research is significantly less well developed than the comparable adult literature (Solomon et al. 1992). From a clinical perspective, we did not find convincing efficacy for any one therapeutic approach for the treatment of child and adolescent PTSD. The next section of this chapter provides conceptual and technical guidance to help structure and focus the treatment activities of clinicians treating traumatized children. It is implied that the guidelines presented here should be considered in the dynamic context of the child's age; modifications must be made to correspond with the child's language ability and more generally his or her developmental context.

A Brief Summary of Studies of Treatment Without Trauma Symptoms as Outcome Measures

The literature includes 10 studies, detailed in Table 5–3, that did not include any measures of trauma symptoms among their outcome measures, yet still focused on the treatment of children exposed to traumatic events. These studies included children who had experienced sexual abuse, physical abuse, bereavement, and natural disasters and who had witnessed domestic violence. Studies on survivors of trauma have detected a high prevalence of PTSD diagnoses. The target symptoms of these studies generally included depression, anxiety, and behavior problems rather than specific trauma symptoms. With regard to these 10 studies, Table 5–4 describes study adherence to the same rigorous standards of methodology used in Table 5–2 and described above.

A comparison of the studies summarized in Tables 5–1 and 5–3 reveals that the studies addressed a differing mix of trauma types. Table 5–1 includes three studies of natural disasters, two studies of sexually abused children, one of mixed trauma, and one of a maritime accident. Table 5–3 includes five studies of sexual abuse, two of natural disaster, one of physical

TABLE 5–3. Studies of traumatic stress without PTSD outcome measure

Study	Treatment description	Subjects	Treatment type/length	Follow-up/time since trauma	Past/concurrent treatment	Findings
Berliner and Saunders 1996	Group CBT with SIT and gradual exposure Controlled comparison	103, sexual abuse 32, index group 48, group CBT 8 boys, 72 girls Mean age, 8 23 dropouts	10 weeks of CBT group therapy, the index group focused on SIT and gradual exposure in some of the sessions.	1 and 2 years/ Not reported	Most children had received between 3–6 individual therapy sessions before referral.	No differences were found between groups regarding improvement of fear (Fear Survey Schedule for Children–Revised; Sexual Abuse Fear Evaluation Scale) and anxiety symptoms (RCMAS).
Cohen and Mannarino 1996, 1997	Individual CBT Controlled randomized	86, sexual abuse 39, CBT 28, supportive therapy 28 boys, 39 girls Mean age, 4.6 19 dropouts	Twelve 90-minute treatment sessions: 50 minutes with parent and 30–40 minutes with child	6 months and 1 year/ Within previous 6 months	Not reported.	CBT group less symptomatic on the Child Sexual Behavior Inventory and Weekly Behavior Record. Also the CBT group mean scores on all measures fell to a nonclinical range (CSB, WBR, and CBCL). Treatment results were maintained at 6 months and 1 year.

TABLE 5–3. Studies of traumatic stress without PTSD outcome measure *(continued)*

Study	Treatment description	Subjects	Treatment type/length	Follow-up/time since trauma	Past/concurrent treatment	Findings
Field et al. 1996	Massage Controlled randomized	60, natural disaster 30, massage 30, video attention 34 boys, 26 girls Mean age, 7.5 No attrition	Compared 30 minutes of back massage to 30 minutes of watching videos, 2 times per week for 4 weeks	None/4 weeks after hurricane	Not reported	After each massage session, decreased state anxiety (State Anxiety Inventory), salivary cortisol and increased Happy Faces Scale. At study end, massage group had decreased anxiety (RCMAS) and depression (CEDS), lower scores on problem behavior, and increased relaxation scores (self drawings and observations).

TABLE 5–3. Studies of traumatic stress without PTSD outcome measure *(continued)*

Study	Treatment description	Subjects	Treatment type/length	Follow-up/time since trauma	Past/concurrent treatment	Findings
Kolko 1996	Individual CBT vs. family therapy (FT) Controlled randomized	55, physical abuse 20, CBT 17, FT 10, routine services 34 boys, 13 girls Mean age, 8.6 8 dropouts	Individual CBT with child and parent vs. FT vs. routine community services (RCS). Twelve 1-hour weekly sessions within 16 weeks	3 months and 6 months/ Within past 6 months	4 children taking medication	Both CBT and FT groups showed significant improvement compared with RCS. No significant differences between CBT and FT; both decreased children's externalizing behavior (CBCL, YSR), general parental distress (Family Environment Scale) and conflict (Conflict Behavior Questionnaire), and increased family cohesion (Parenting Scale).
Tonkins and Lambert 1996	Group CBT Controlled comparison	22, bereavement 16, CBT 6, control 10 boys, 12 girls Mean age, 9.1	8-week CBT grief therapy group	None/ Within past year	Not reported	CBT group showed significant decrease in sadness, anger, withdrawal, guilt, anxiety, loneliness, helplessness, (all CBCL, TRF) and depression (CDI).

TABLE 5–3. Studies of traumatic stress without PTSD outcome measure (*continued*)

Study	Treatment description	Subjects	Treatment type/length	Follow-up/time since trauma	Past/concurrent treatment	Findings
McGain and McKinzey 1995	Group CBT Controlled comparison	30, sexual abuse 15, group CBT 15, control 30 girls Mean age, 10.5 Attrition not reported	Once a week for a total of 9–12 months of group CBT	None/ Within 1 year	Not reported.	60%–100% of all participants had abnormal scores on the Quay Revised Behavioral Problem Checklist and Eyberg Child Behavior Inventory. After treatment, 0%–33% of treatment group showed abnormal scores whereas 60%–100% of control group continue to have abnormal scores.

TABLE 5–3. Studies of traumatic stress without PTSD outcome measure *(continued)*

Study	Treatment description	Subjects	Treatment type/length	Follow-up/time since trauma	Past/concurrent treatment	Findings
Wagar and Rodway 1995	Group CBT Controlled randomized	42, witness to domestic violence 16, group CBT 22, control 26 boys, 12 girls Mean age, 10 4 dropouts	10-week group CBT.	None/ 3 months violence free period	Not reported.	CBT group showed sig. decrease in attitudes and responses to anger (Conflict Tactics Scale) and sense of responsibility for the parents and for the violence (Child Witness to Violence Questionnaire). No sig. difference between groups on sense of safety and support skills.
Sullivan et al. 1992	Individual CBT/ Supportive Controlled comparison	72, sexual abuse 35, CBT 37, control 51 boys, 21 girls Age, 12–16 No attrition	2 hours of individual CBT/supportive therapy per week for 36 weeks.	None/Not reported	All children were residents at a school for the deaf. Control group were sexually abused; however, parents refused treatment.	Children receiving therapy had significantly fewer behavior problems than control group based on CBCL scores.

TABLE 5–3.   Studies of traumatic stress without PTSD outcome measure (*continued*)

Study	Treatment description	Subjects	Treatment type/length	Follow-up/time since trauma	Past/concurrent treatment	Findings
Galante and Foa 1986	Group CBT Controlled comparison	300, natural disaster 62, CBT 238, control 1st–4th grades No attrition	Seven CBT group treatment sessions met 1 hour over 1 academic year approximately monthly	None/6 months	Not reported	There was a greater reduction of at-risk scores (Rutter Behavioral Questionnaire for Completion by Teachers) in children who had been in the treatment program.
Verleur et al. 1986	Supportive group plus sex education Controlled comparison	30, sexual abuse 15, group therapy 15, control 30 girls Age, 13–17 Attrition not reported	Supportive female-led group therapy with sexual education, weekly for 6 months	None/Not reported	All were in a residential facility and received milieu therapy offered at the facility	Group therapy participants showed significant increase in self-esteem (Coopersmith Self-Esteem Inventory) and increased knowledge of human sexuality, birth control, and venereal disease (Anatomy/Physiology Sexual Awareness Scale).

Note.   CBT=cognitive-behavioral therapy; CES-D=Center for Epidemiological Studies Depression Scale; CSBI=Child Sexual Behavior Inventory; CBCL=Child Behavior Checklist; RCMAS=Revised Children's Manifest Anxiety Scale; SIT=Stress Inoculation Training; TRF=Teacher Report Form; WBR=Weekly Behavior Report; YSR=Youth Self Report.

TABLE 5–4. Gold standards for treatment outcome: studies without traumatic stress outcome measures

Study	PTSD or trauma symptoms	Clearly defined target symptoms	Reliable valid measures	Blind evaluators	Assessor training	Manualized replicable specific treatment	Random assignment	Treatment adherence
Berliner and Saunders 1996	No	Yes	Yes	Yes	Not reported	Yes	Yes	Yes
Cohen and Mannarino 1996, 1997	No	No	Yes	Not clear	Not reported	Yes	Yes	Yes
Field et al. 1996	PTSD, only pretreatment	Yes	Yes	Yes	Not reported	No	Yes	No
Kolko 1996	No	No	Yes	Yes	Not reported	Yes	Yes	Yes
Tonkins and Lambert 1996	No	No	No	No	Not reported	Yes	No	No
McGain and McKinzey 1995	No	No	Yes	No	Not reported	Not reported	No	Not reported
Wagar and Rodway 1995	No	Yes	No	No	Not reported	Yes	Yes	Not reported
Sullivan et al. 1992	No	No	Yes	Yes	Not reported	No	No	No
Galante and Foa 1986	No	Yes	Yes	Yes	Not reported	Not reported	No	No
Verleur et al. 1986	No	Yes	No	Not reported	Not reported	No	Not reported	Not reported

abuse, one of bereavement, and one of witnesses to violence. The major difference is that Table 5–1 includes primarily natural disaster studies and Table 5–3 primarily sexual abuse studies. At this time, it appears that treatment research for victims of sexual and physical abuse, which usually involves multiple traumatization and a complex medicolegal environment, is not as well advanced as research on single major traumatic events, such as natural disasters.

A Conceptual and Practical Framework to Guide Single-Event Child Trauma Treatment

In this section, our conceptual perspective and a practical description of our clinical approach to single-event trauma in children are briefly presented to inform clinicians beyond what is generally presented in empirical reports of research. It should be highlighted that given the current level of knowledge, this information is presented as a heuristic starting point for less experienced child trauma clinicians and as a reference to provoke comparison between the clinical approaches used by more experienced clinicians. This chapter does not address the treatment of recurrent trauma by family members. Such traumas differ from the impact of single-event trauma in two major ways. First, the regulation of safety in children is based on the core biological assumption that one's caretaker can be trusted, and that the "enemy" comes from without (typically a predator). When the "predator" is a close family member the distinction between self (friend) and not-self (not-friend/predator), which is at the core of the management of personal safety, becomes profoundly confused. This can affect the normal development of cognitive structures that support both the management of safety and the process of individuation in the child. Consequently, the sensitive treatment of such traumas represents a major challenge to clinicians. The problems associated with the treatment of such traumas are sufficiently distinct from the treatment of single-event trauma that they fall beyond the scope of this chapter.

Events that are potentially traumatic are defined in DSM-IV as involving actual or threatened death or serious injury, either to one's self or to significant others. Furthermore, the prospect of death or injury must provoke intense fear, helplessness, or horror. As such, these types of events obviously directly affect the ongoing sense of psychological safety, even as they serve to mobilize automatic psychological processes that support survival in the face of threat.

Where children are concerned, the experience of safety is inextricably bound up not only in the self, but also in the children's perception of the safety and competence of caretakers. Moreover, in most circumstances the same events that threatened the child are also likely to have threatened his or her caretakers. For example, children exposed to disasters or to automobile accidents are usually so exposed while in the company of caretakers. This means that restoring a sense of safety to children usually requires addressing the experience of both child and parent or caretaker. This is one critical way in which children differ from adults and even older adolescents.

Clearly, the youngest children experience most intensely this sense of shared identity in the context of danger. Indeed, in very young infants the traumatic event is experienced primarily through its impact on the relational context that protects the infant. Barring direct physical injury, the very young child is traumatized in large measure because of the impact of the trauma on those charged with maintaining his or her physical and psychological safety. Thus, this perspective requires considering the child as operating both subjectively and descriptively within a broader psychological system that serves to maintain and regulate psychological safety. The most effective interventions are those that recognize that trauma disrupts this adaptively embedded quality of the child's experience and seek to restore its functionality.

The effective treatment of traumatized children requires us to understand how the sense of psychological safety is affected in children. The most significant factor is the automatic activation of specialized information processing mechanisms that assist the person in dealing with danger. We have previously described this as the activation of a "survival mode" of functioning (Chemtob et al. 1988). This model, unlike pathology-based models, focuses attention on the evolution of specialized information processing mechanisms that support an organism's response to threat. PTSD and trauma are proposed to reflect a lowered threshold for the activation of "survival-mode" functioning.

Survival mode may be characterized as reflecting the "emergency" response of people. Just as animals faced with predator threat respond in relatively stereotypical ways, we have proposed that individuals as well, when faced with threat, react in "prepared" ways rooted in evolution that are specialized to support surviving threats.

Survival mode is automatically activated by evidence of life threat and preempts normal modes of response. When in survival mode, people respond more rigidly and their behavioral repertoire is less flexible. This does not reflect mere "regression" but rather the activation of information structures that are specialized for threat processing. Such specialization has the virtue of increased response speed and decreased dithering. However, once survival mode is activated, nonthreat information is processed as reflecting on survival. That is, once survival mode is activated via confirmation biases, information about threat leads to active seeking of confirming evidence of threat.

The activation of survival mode often induces a sense of identity fragmentation, as most people identify themselves with the continuity of their experience in normal "safe" circumstances. This automaticity is also disruptive of normal functioning because it means an increased fragmentation in the sense of self between normal functioning and the decreased posttraumatic threshold to shift into survival mode. An additional important characteristic of survival mode activation is that by virtue of focusing resources on threat processing, self-monitoring is significantly reduced. As a consequence of the loss of self-monitoring and the automaticity of survival-mode activation, people do not necessarily recognize that they are operating in survival mode.

We have further proposed that in human beings survival mode incorporates two specific survival subsystems, a threat detection system and an attachment system. The threat detection system has developed to efficiently acquire information about threat and risk in the environment. Its activation entrains a bias to perceive danger in the environment, global (gestalt) processing, a lowered threshold for responding to evidence of threat (which can be misperceived as generalized impulsivity), and multimodal information processing. This means physiologic arousal, sensory information, and cognitive expectations are all integrated in a positive-feedback bias (confirmatory bias). Partial information of threat from multiple channels is sufficient to activate the organism's emergency response.

The attachment system has been relatively neglected in research on adult PTSD. However, it is central in the survival response of children. The attachment system reflects the fact that we are social animals whose inclusion in a social group determines our survival. Thus, when faced by threats we immediately assess not only where and what the threat is (where the predator or enemy is) but also who is on "our side" and who is "against us." In sum, concerns about social inclusion and exclusion reflect calculations about one's strength relative to the threat and take into account support from one's "extended social self" as a critical resource.

We have proposed that normal relationship modes are organized differently in threat contexts. For example, warriors in battle form extraordinary personal bonds that sustain their effective action and increase their personal chances of survival. Similarly, in disaster circumstances, people experience automatic nonconscious increases in altruism and in feeling that "everyone is in the same boat." This automatic activation of powerful kinship feelings leads to increased social cohesion, increased social support, and increased cooperation at the time it is most needed. The distinction between what is "mine" and what is "yours" appears to be diminished during times of disaster, reflecting shifts in the relative fluidity of the self-other boundary. It should be recalled that these shifts in the mode of attachment are activated automatically and with a loss of self-monitoring as part of the activation of survival mode.

Relatively little is known about these structured survival programs in children. However, the research programs stimulated by Bowlby's (1988) seminal contribution have focused our attention on the importance of specialized psychobiological mechanisms in children that have evolved to regulate their sense of safety through monitoring their distance from their mother. In this regard, the important theoretical work that has tied psychological individuation and separation to the capacity to regulate proximity and separation is extremely important in guiding the child trauma therapist. In effect, this work highlights that psychological safety is maintained and developed by anchoring safety through maintaining a tie to a caretaking other. The purpose of exploration becomes the development of increased capacity to maintain individuated safety. Conversely, with development comes increased capacity for flexible exploration. One has only to examine a child who is exploring the environment (while keeping tabs on his mother) and becomes frightened to understand the impact of threat on traumatized children. The child's reaction is almost universally to retreat in alarm to the mother. Thereafter, the child becomes substantially more cautious in exploration and retreats back to the mother in reaction to "evidence" of threat that previously would have been insufficient to qualify as threatening. This lowered threshold for accepting information as evidence of threat obviously interferes with the activation of processes that would otherwise promote a sense of safety.

The clinician's task is to actively help the child intrude on the automatic activation of survival mode by restoring his or her capacity to evaluate the presence of threat. This is done by supporting the restoration of regulatory capacity. The child must be aided in reacquiring skills for regulating arousal, for making exploratory cognitive assessments, and for maintaining an individuated self, all such skills being naturally compromised by the automatic activation of survival mode. In cases where children never acquired the requisite skills to maintain age-appropriate psychological safety, these skills must be taught for the first time. In this latter case it is necessary to reverse the interference of trauma with the normal developmental process, the process in which increasingly sophisticated self-regulatory skills are acquired to support safety.

Role of the Therapist

Multiple root metaphors inform the actions of trauma therapists. These usually reflect particular theoretical models of etiology. We believe that these metaphors are largely complementary. The challenge for therapists is 1) to consistently apply them at the right time and in the right context, 2) to avoid mistaking a part of the function of treatment for the whole, and 3) to use multiple treatment means to achieve a clearly articulated therapeutic aim, focused on clearly specified treatment targets.

For example, one of the earliest metaphors incorporated in psychotherapeutic practice is that of catharsis. This metaphor was rooted in the proposition that psychological discharge is akin to the discharge of a reflex. It was thought that once discharged, the dissipation of "blocked" psychological energy would result in resolution of the problematic symptom. This is implicit in the actions of therapists who invite their patients to cry or "let it all out." In fact, this metaphor is a double-edged sword. Simply expressing one's feelings can in fact be re-traumatizing. The expression of feeling while mobilizing memories of a traumatic event does not necessarily resolve the psychological experience.

A more modern elaboration of the catharsis proposition is the notion that the construction of a cohesive narrative representing an otherwise fragmentary experience permits the elaboration of more adaptive representations of events. Thus, the emotional reworking of a traumatic memory in the course of elaborating a more complex representation of the event incorporates corrective information about the experience. This reworked and elaborated representation has different psychological characteristics that permit a more adaptive (less rigid) set of responses to the traumatic event. Our approach differs from this in putting the emphasis on the release of evolutionary structures specially suited for threat response from regulatory control when faced with a life-threat. The subsequent facilitation of activation of survival mode is incompatible with the activation of regulatory processes that sustain psychological safety. Thus, rather than merely seeking assimilation of the experience, we seek to restore and teach the skills that permit the traumatized child to suppress the context-inappropriate activation of survival mode.

Another treatment metaphor regarding trauma originates in learning-theory models of the etiology of phobic disorders. In such models, it is assumed that there is a failure to incorporate corrective information about the phobic object because avoidance drives the fearful person away from contact with the fear-provoking stimuli. This avoidance therefore interferes with normal learning about the realistic characteristics of the feared object. Although it appears that exposure to traumatic events is an important component of effective trauma treatment, it is not clear whether it is the exposure component or the support of a responsive therapist in the context of exposure that is effective. Moreover, the learning-theory approach generally tends to underestimate the importance of evolutionary mechanisms in the genesis of psychopathology, particularly trauma-related pathology.

We believe that much of the apparent effectiveness of exposure is not due to exposure per se but rather to the support of a trusted therapist who serves as an external regulatory support, permitting the patient to have an increased capacity to master an otherwise frightening and overwhelming reactivation of the traumatic experience. Consequently, we put the emphasis in using therapeutic exposure on empathic management of dosage. The dose of exposure should be used much like weights are used by physical therapists engaged in muscle rehabilitation. The dose of exposure should never exceed the ability of the child to feel mastery, while requiring an effort just beyond what the child might have undertaken without the encouragement and skilled guidance of a therapist. Our emphasis therefore is on supported and sustained practice of regulatory skills in the face of the challenge of exposure.

Thus, the treatment perspective we prefer, and which we believe has been largely neglected in this field, is that trauma treatment is rehabilitative. Its purpose is to support restoring self-regulatory skills that maintain psychological safety when such skills are suppressed by trauma-related facilitation of survival responses. Moreover, we believe that in children (and adults) the treatment of trauma is often habilitative. It must specifically support acquiring age-appropriate self-regulation skills when fundamental psychological skills were never acquired because trauma interrupted or distorted the normal processes of skill acquisition.

Treating Single-Event Trauma

Clinic-Based Approach

Among single-event traumas are motor vehicle accidents, animal attacks, exposure to domestic and community violence, physical assault, and other life-threatening experiences. Children who experience single events that are traumatic often present for treatment in traditional clinical settings, whether this be an individual practitioner's office or a hospital- or clinic-based practice. However, presenting because of a dramatic single event does not in and of itself permit ruling out a history of chronic victimization. Clinicians should recognize that such chronic victimization, for example, sexual or physical abuse, may not only constitute part of the pretrauma environment but may also be ongoing. Therefore, a complete trauma history should be obtained as part of an initial assessment.

In treating traumatized children, the clinician must recognize that the trauma of children affects both the child and the caretaking system in which the child is embedded. Parents and caretakers are directly affected by the trauma in cases where they are exposed to it at the same time as the child. On an indirect level, they are affected because the suffering of one's child can mobilize extremely strong realistic and unrealistic reactions. As trauma interferes with the child's regulatory operations that sustain a sense of psychological safety, parents and caretakers can be emotionally reactive, making it difficult for the child to reestablish self-regulation. Their own symptoms can interfere with empathy and psychological availability to their child, rendering them ineffective in modulating the child's increased reactivity. An overanxious parent will not be resilient when the child's withdrawal, either through overt hostility or covert avoidance, engenders feelings of rejection in the parent. Consequently, involvement and education of parents in the treatment of traumatized children is critical.

In the ideal treatment situation, the therapist must not only educate parents as to the particular treatment needs of their child but must also educate parents so that they understand the normative (what is to be expected) effects of trauma. This will hopefully enable parents to avoid overpersonalizing their child's reactions and instead allow them to provide an environment capable of supporting regaining safety. In addition, it is clearly important that parents be taught specific techniques to help the child gain mastery over the trauma experience. Parents must also be provided with the assurance that the therapist will support them throughout the recovery process. This will enable the parents to be more resilient and flexible in the face of the helplessness that their child's pain engenders. Furthermore, this increased resilience will permit the therapist to tactfully explore the impact of the traumatic event on the parents. In doing so, it is extremely important to treat parental reactions as reflecting positive attempts at caregiving. For example, guilt that one did not prevent child victimization should be reframed as evidence of concern and responsibility.

Children also benefit from age-appropriate education regarding their experience. Key elements of this education include reassurance that 1) other children have had such experiences and have gotten to feel better, 2) the doctor has helped other children with similar problems and can help the child get better, and 3), the doctor can tolerate and absorb the wide variety of feelings that the child might feel toward him or her. Recognition of this last factor is particularly important because expressing negative feelings (anger, disappointment, betrayal) toward parents (a major source of safety) can be extremely threatening to the child who may fear that such expressions might cause rejection by his or her parents.

In working with older children it can be very useful to explain the therapist's role as being akin to that of a special teacher who is an expert in teaching children about horrible experiences. This permits the therapist to take on a supportive coaching role that is familiar to many children. Clarifying the role of the therapist reduces ambiguity about the roles of each participant and is therefore supportive, increasing the child's sense of competence and therefore safety. Failing to clarify the purpose of therapy, and the role of the therapist, sometimes leads to the child perceiving the therapist as dangerous, and even as an enemy, "unnecessarily digging up the painful past," which is better left alone.

A critical first step for successful treatment is the specific assessment of a child's capacity to maintain a treatment relationship in the face of threat activation. Threat activation affects the relationship of the child to caregiving adults. Typically, a child faced with threat and reminders of the trauma will react either by clinging to adults for safety or by withdrawing from contact. Clinging interferes with a range of ego functions such as exploration and the establishment of autonomous identity. Specifically, it interferes with any activity by the therapist that seeks to support the child's independence, as such activities are experienced as threatening to the child's sense of being protected. Conversely, children who are withdrawn typically have concluded that they cannot rely on the protection of adults and therefore become difficult to make contact with, which includes difficulty in maintaining a treatment alliance. In both instances, what has occurred is an increased rigidity in relationships with caretakers that interferes with the flexible exploration and rapprochement that are hallmarks of healthy relationships with adult caretakers. The therapist's task is to focus quite explicitly (though usually in displacement) through the medium of play, drawing, and the like, on the relationship of the child to the therapist. Themes of strength versus weakness, of curiosity versus hiding, and of trust versus betrayal usually dominate this aspect of treatment. For example, a child who has been severely bitten by a dog will often feel betrayed by parental caretakers. Simultaneously, he or she will exhibit fluctuations between feeling strong and feeling weak, which will usually be exaggerated. And there will be concerns about trusting adults concurrent with trusting animals. Reenacting these concerns with the therapist through the medium of play addresses specific trauma symptoms and their deeper impact on the child's capacity to relate to adults effectively.

Although one can expect that the core response to trauma will involve similar major components among most children, each child lives that aspect of the trauma in a highly distinct and personal way. Generally, single-event traumas seem to affect four dimensions. The initial impact usually involves shock, disbelief, and a sense of helplessness, expressing itself around themes of vulnerability and abandonment. The second issue to emerge usually involves losses experienced by the child as a result of victimization. This can be highly specific ("my kitty cat died") or quite general ("I am sad"). Third, anger and scapegoating are often expressed both as a defense against the sadness and as a primary affect reflecting mobilization to address recovery. Finally, as recovery proceeds successfully, one often observes the child struggling to create new capacities for coping based on working through the trauma. These generic steps on the way to psychological recovery are modified by the particular characteristics of specific traumatic events. For this reason, inexperienced trauma therapists would do well to consult more experienced therapists who have greater knowledge of the common aftereffects of particular trauma.

There are a number of aspects of each trauma that must be explored. These include the impact of the trauma on cognition, on affect and arousal, on the mode of relationship (attachment), and on the child's sense of identity. The theme of safety versus feeling unsafe or threatened provides the common lens through which to explore these issues. This analysis should be done in the form of reconstructing the experience, beginning with what was going on well before the trauma took place. Such exploration is a key part of the actual treatment because it recapitulates the experience in detail while assisting the child to reestablish a capacity to create a cohesive narrative. We emphasize that this narrative is defined not only by talking, but rather mostly by drawing, playing, play-acting, and a wide variety of other child therapy techniques.

Because the recollection of traumatic experiences is so compelling, it tends to weaken a child's sense of what is past and what is present. Restoring such clear temporal articulation is an important goal of treatment. The therapist's support enables the child to reframe his or her experience by maintaining, side by side, a representation of the traumatic experience (with all its impacts) that is linked to the past, with a representation of safety that relates to the present. In this regard, it is critical to always weave into the treatment a clear differentiation between what happened in the past and what is occurring in the present. In providing the child with the necessary support so he or she can ultimately relive the traumatic experience from a position of mastery, it is also important to teach the child to monitor his or her internal states to anticipate being overwhelmed by reminders of the traumatic experience.

In exploring the impact of trauma on cognition, it is cleat that, as with adults, trauma induces cognitive deficits in children. These deficits, not usually recognized as taking place because of trauma-induced loss of self-monitoring, include a heightened sense that dangerous events are probable and a tendency to proactively color experiences as being more negative. There is often a tendency to interpret events using a global frame of reference, which can lead to missing either disconfirming cues or cues of actual danger. Also, dissociative cognitive styles can emerge that are expressed as cognitive avoidance. These cognitive deficits can lead to the child being less competent in judging threat. As cognitive deficits are identified, and the child is helped to recognize them, a skill-building approach aimed at increasing the child's cognitive competence in the face of threat activation is very useful. The therapist can use play in rebuilding the child's skill, which itself induces a different shared frame of reference regarding the trauma.

The impact of trauma on affect and arousal is an area that defines yet another task of the therapist, that of helping the child to reestablish or gain skills in the modulation of affect and arousal. When faced with threat, affect takes on considerable primacy in orienting the child to the danger and in guiding an effective adaptive response. In the posttraumatic context, the reaction to events that activate a sense of threat tends to be characterized by affective primacy. The child reads the intensity of reaction as representing confirmation that the situation is unsafe. This confirmatory bias acts as a positive feedback loop, threat activation inducing affective reaction and arousal, further confirming threat. Because of the lack of self-monitoring, this feedback increases the intensity of affect and arousal without inducing a regulatory cognitive response ("I am overreacting; this is safe"). The role of treatment is to reestablish the ability to self-monitor the automatic activation of affect and arousal and to support the establishment of coping responses (seeking help from a grownup, drawing feelings, breathing deeply, thinking about what to do) that are incompatible with reacting automatically to threat.

The experience of trauma has been linked to the automatic activation of survival mode, which in turn affects a child's sense of self-cohesion and identity. The reaction to threat preempts other processing, contributing to the sense that the child's reaction has a life of its own. Traumatized children are repeatedly set off into survival mode (the threshold for perceiving the presence of threat is lowered), which creates discontinuity in their sense of identity. Consequently, the child often feels a degree of dissociation from his or her normal sense of self. The reactions and thoughts that are familiar points of self-reference are replaced with relatively rigid responses that serve to facilitate survival. This sense of self-fragmentation itself decreases feelings of safety. Part of the task of treatment in this regard is to explain to the child the nature of a survival reaction, thus restoring a sense of continuity in the child's sense of self. Obviously, this occurs primarily through play, play-acting, and other metaphorical modes of communication. For example, it is sometimes helpful to play with the child (either directly or in displacement through the use of drawings or puppets) at being an animal, peacefully minding his or her business, that gets surprised or frightened by a threatening other animal. The therapist then notes the difference between how the animal acts and feels when peaceful and when threatened.

This contrast permits heightening both the contrast between the two modes of response and the fact that they are responses emitted by the same animal.

The purpose of exposure in dealing with cognitive effects, affect and arousal, attachment, and sense of identity is primarily to reactivate the child's threat response. As noted above, we do not believe that exposure on its own is sufficient. Indeed, it is often so upsetting to both child and parent that it can engender treatment avoidance and premature treatment termination. Rather, dosed exposure is most useful as a means to intensify the components of the child's threat response so that they can be mastered bit by bit. When dosed exposure is used, this permits educating the child regarding the various components of the child's thoughts, feelings, and actions when provoked into survival mode. As each of these components is identified, the child is first taught to self-monitor these components of his or her reactions and then is taught to interrupt these reactions by activating responses incompatible with survival mode. This serves to restore increased mastery and flexibility in the child's repertoire.

The final phase of treatment establishes skills necessary to care for oneself in the future if faced with similar threats. Often, this can be accomplished by putting the child in the role of "teacher" to other (usually) imaginary children regarding his or her traumatic experience and the methods of coping with it. The emphasis in this phase of treatment is teaching the child to distinguish between feeling safe and feeling realistically threatened. The child is helped to anticipate such situations and to rehearse coping scenarios using a stress inoculation framework.

Community- and School-Based Approaches

In contrast to children who present in clinical practice one at a time, natural disasters, technological disasters, or other large-scale events usually involve a large number of potentially affected children. Because of the numbers involved, clinicians are called on to use different strategic models to guide their interventions. Guidelines for these types of events are presented below. In instances of disaster, therapists should recognize that they must adapt their interventions in different ways during different phases of disaster recovery. One can conceptualize the phases of disaster impact as preimpact; during impact; and immediate, early, middle, and late disaster recovery. Consequently, it should be obvious that interventions intended to support traumatized children must be appropriate to the needs of each period.

In this regard, a public health perspective is a useful framework to guide clinicians. In the preimpact period, educating communities and supporting planning for coordinated disaster management is akin to primary prevention. In this way, the primary systems that affect children (schools, parents and caretakers, media, disaster authorities) will be better able to mobilize during a disaster and to act in coordinated ways that are sensitive to the needs of children, thus reducing the likelihood of psychological morbidity. Hopefully, such preparation will yield effective intervention during the actual impact phase. Unfortunately, resources to support psychological recovery usually are not deployed until after the fact. It therefore behooves clinicians to proactively pursue integration of knowledge about the psychological impact of disaster on children in school disaster planning and in community disaster planning efforts. Authorities will usually welcome offers of proactive support, together with education about its importance. Proactive planning leads to building working relationships before the disaster's impact. As a result, when disasters do strike, it is easier to enlist cooperation based on preexisting working relationships.

Because natural disasters often affect the community's infrastructure and lead to evacuation to safe areas, early postdisaster intervention will generally occur in the context of community shelters (interestingly, schools are often designated as such shelters). In such instances, one is not directly treating PTSD but rather is providing psychosocial support to assist parents and others in the care of their children. Such early interventions are intended to augment the natural capacities of parents to maintain their children's psychological safety in the context of a threat. It is assumed that such early intervention is reassuring and supportive and may help prevent the later development of PTSD. However, the latter assumption has not been empirically evaluated as yet.

Immediately following the active phase of the disaster (e.g., after the hurricane or after the major shocks of an earthquake), clinicians will typically continue to provide education and reassurance through communal channels (e.g., relief/assistance lines), to provide practical training to paraprofessionals and others involved in the recovery effort, and to engage available media resources in an effort to provide information regarding children's normative reactions. Such community education provides reassurance to parents by indicating the normative characteristics of postdisaster psychological reactions; increases community capacity to maintain safety; and provides referral sources for situations when it is appropriate to seek outside assistance for children. An additional role for more senior and experienced trauma clinicians is to serve as consultants to the civil authorities regarding community psychological concerns and to help the individuals responsible for managing the crises in dealing with the extraordinary stresses imposed by large-scale disaster recovery efforts.

Early efforts to assist in the children's psychological recovery from disaster usually begin with the reopening of schools, the timing of which is itself a sensitive issue. In determining the appropriate time to reopen a school, the need to restore predictable order in the lives of children and to provide a structure for the safekeeping of children while freeing adults to tend to recovery tasks must be balanced with the recognition that teachers and other school personnel have themselves been affected by the disaster. Opening schools too early can leave teachers feeling as if their needs are not considered important. Conversely, delaying school opening impairs community recovery. Clinicians who operate in a postdisaster environment will often be asked to advise on the timing of school reopening. Their role in this regard should be to clarify the psychological component of the decision and to be advocates for maintaining flexibility. In my (CMC) experience, reopening schools as soon as possible is effective when coupled with explicit provisions permitting flexibility for school personnel to determine their ability to return to school. School administrators should be made aware that divisiveness could result among administrators and personnel based on how this decision is managed. Moreover, the decision will be evaluated in the context of biases perceived as already existing among top officials and principals. Thus, for example, if a school administrator is viewed as being too concerned about public opinion, early reopening will tend to be perceived as further evidence of caring more about public opinion than about staff. This confirmatory bias can complicate recovery efforts by creating divisive factionalism.

Clinicians who have established predisaster relationships with top school officials will find it much easier to work in schools once a disaster actually occurs. Failing such preparation, it is important to understand that schools are normally vigilant about letting outsiders in. Whereas this is usually relaxed during crises, it remains extremely important to develop collaborative relationships with key people who are highly respected and can provide credibility internally as well as prevent cultural missteps by outsiders. Such partners can make it possible to recruit a far higher level of cooperation with psychological interventions.

In the early phase of school-based intervention, a number of models have been used that are all largely derived from psychological debriefing models. For example, certain school districts such as the Los Angeles Unified School District have developed debriefing models that involve up to several hundred students working through the aftereffects of a catastrophic experience. More frequently, clinicians use the individual classroom as a locus of intervention, sometimes collaborating with the classroom teacher, sometimes merely having the classroom teacher in the classroom to ensure cooperation from children. Others have provided school counselors with brief specialized training and relied on their established relationships with teachers and students to maximize the effect of the intervention.

Generally, all the interventions have as a common goal helping students create a coherent cognitive map of the events that transpired, generating support to assist students in dealing with the shock of the experience and in managing loss, and assisting children in generating positive coping responses. Remarkably, given that many now consider this type of support a standard of practice, we are aware of no published data demonstrating that these activities are really helpful to students. However, they certainly reduce the sense of helplessness among adults. Our approach is to proceed on multiple fronts. We generally seek to provide training for school counselors and key administrators (principals, vice principals) to increase the capacity within schools to manage the aftereffects of the disaster. We typically also provide an experience that joins elements of group debriefing with education for teachers to assist them in understanding their own experience as a prelude to helping learn how to assist their students' needs. An important part of the training is to help the adults recognize the symptoms that can characterize children whose recovery does not proceed apace. In relatively few instances, we have been able to provide information to parents. More often, we send an informational letter or brochure to parents to alert them to the nature of normative responses to disaster among children.

Relatively recently, a number of clinicians have recognized that disaster recovery takes substantially longer than had been previously thought. Because federal assistance dollars are usually provided for no more than a year, there has been a tendency to align activities to support the recovery of children to the period of time in which funding is available. This early phase of recovery is the easiest, because during this time most people experience distress and are therefore available to help each other. However, as time passes and exhaustion sets in, trauma victims—and children in particular—who continue to experience disaster-related trauma symptoms begin to be circumspect about admitting their continued distress. Children often acknowledge the burdens placed on their parents and prefer to keep their own symptoms hidden for fear of overtaxing their parents. As a result of this middisaster dynamic, it becomes important to use strategies that rely on large-scale screening of children for trauma symptoms. In our own work, we elected to screen children across an entire school district. We then provided trauma-specific treatment to the children with the highest level of trauma symptoms. We used specially trained counselors to provide treatment that was conceptualized as secondary prevention. Specifically, we sought to mobilize the children's own recovery capacity. Although our treatment did improve symptoms, the effect sizes were quite modest. This may have been accounted for by the fact that although most students got better after treatment, some did not improve and some got worse. Our follow-up study using EMDR and trained doctoral-level clinicians yielded substantially larger effect sizes. This reopens the question of whether one should use doctoral-level clinicians from the outset and encourages further evaluation of EMDR for postdisaster treatment. For greater detail regarding our approach to middisaster recovery, please see Chemtob et al. (1999) and Chemtob et al. (in press).

The final stage of supporting postdisaster recovery requires assisting the school community to generate something new, of value, produced as a result of the disaster. It is important to do so in order that the memories of the disaster are capped by a positive achievement, symbolizing the capacity of the community to create something positive out of the hardships of the disaster. An example from our work on Kauai may clarify this point. On Kauai, one valuable lesson learned in the schools after the disaster is that schools need to be more welcoming to "outsider" child helpers such as psychologists than they had been under normal circumstances. After the early phases of the disaster recovery process, the schools sought out additional help for children who were still having difficulty. This new school openness led to the formulation of a new plan on Kauai that restructured and greatly expanded mental health services to a school-based mental health system. After the disaster, and after much struggle, the Kauai school system was able to create mental health clinics in each of the Kauai schools. The schools' community united to advocate for a substantial increase in mental health resources. As a result, the island saw mental health resources increase from 1 psychologist to 15 psychologists and from 10 social workers to 22 and saw a doubling of child psychiatrist resources. The island's school-based child mental health system has become the model for the State of Hawaii. This is a source of pride and increased community cohesion for parents, teachers, and professionals alike. Most important, it represents a lasting contribution to the welfare of children in this island community that would not have been created had the community not mobilized effectively to care for its disaster-affected children.

Looking Forward

It is clear that knowledge of the treatment of traumatized children lags well behind the knowledge of adult trauma treatment. This is largely because the field has not engaged in the same systematic research evaluating the nature of the consequences of trauma in children that has been undertaken with adults. Although there is increasing enthusiasm among clinicians to diagnose PTSD in children, many trauma clinicians continue to express concern regarding whether the PTSD diagnosis, derived for adults, accurately fits the clinical phenomenology of traumatized children. To begin to address this critical issue, it is necessary to conduct prospective studies of children exposed to traumatic events to empirically characterize the type, frequency, and patterning of posttraumatic symptoms in children.

Much research on trauma and PTSD in the last 20 years has focused on fear-related systems of response. This is appropriate for many types of adult trauma. However, as noted above, psychological safety in children is mediated in a much larger part through the attachment system. There is a clear need to develop theories of trauma that take this into account. As the specific impacts of trauma on attachment are further clarified, specific treatments can be developed and evaluated that address these consequences in focused and effective ways. The ultimate promise of improving the understanding of trauma treatment in children is that it will increase the understanding of the ways in which developmental vicissitudes and trauma influence children and also the child still present in every adult.

References

Achenbach TM: Manual for the Child Behavior Checklist/4-18 and 1991 Profile. Burlington, VT, University of Vermont, 1991

Achenbach TM, Edelbrock C: Manual for the Child Behavior Checklist and Revised Child Behavior Profile. Burlington, VT, University of Vermont, 1991

American Psychiatric Association: Diagnostic and Statistical Manual of Mental Disorders, 4th Edition. Washington, DC, American Psychiatric Association, 1994

Applebaum DR, Burns GL: Unexpected childhood death: posttraumatic stress disorder in surviving siblings and parents. J Clin Child Psychol 20(2):114–120, 1991

Asarnow JR, Carlson GA: Depression Self-Rating Scale: utility with child psychiatric inpatients. J Consult Clin Psychol 53:491–499, 1985

Berliner L, Saunders BE: Treating fear and anxiety in sexually abused children: results of a controlled 2-year follow-up study. Child Maltreatment 1(4):294–309, 1996

Birleson P: The validity of depressive disorder in childhood and the development of a self-rating scale. J Child Psychol Psychiatry 22:73–88, 1981

Bowlby J: A secure base: parent-child attachment and healthy human development. New York, Basic Books, 1988

Celano M, Hazzard A, Webb C, et al: Treatment of traumagenic beliefs among sexually abused girls and their mothers: an evaluation study. J Abnorm Child Psychol 24(1):1–17, 1996

Chambers WJ, Puig-Antich J, Hirsch M, et al: The assessment of affective disorders in children and adolescents by semistructured interview: test-retest reliability of the Schedule for Affective Disorders and Schizophrenia for School-Age Children, Present Episode Version. Arch Gen Psychiatry 42:696–702, 1985

Chemtob CM, Roitblat HL, Hamada RS, et al: A cognitive action theory of post-traumatic stress disorder. J Anxiety Disord 2:253–275, 1988

Chemtob CM, Nakashima J, Hamada RS, et al: Eye movement desensitization and reprocessing (EMDR) treatment for elementary school children with disaster-related posttraumatic stress disorder: a controlled field study. J Clin Psychol 58(1):99–112, 2002

Chemtob CM, Nakashima JP, Hamada RS: Psychosocial intervention for post-disaster trauma symptoms in elementary school children: a controlled community field study. Arch Pediatr Adolesc Med (in press)

Cohen JA, Mannarino AP: A treatment outcome study for sexually abused preschool children: initial findings. J Am Acad Child Adolesc Psychiatry 35(1):42–50, 1996

Cohen JA, Mannarino AP: A treatment study for sexually abused preschool children: outcome during a one-year follow-up. J Am Acad Child Adolesc Psychiatry 36(9):1228–1235, 1997

Conners CK: A teacher rating scale for use in drug studies with children. Am J Psychiatry 126:884–888, 1969

Deblinger E, McLeer SV, Atkins MS, et al: Posttraumatic stress in sexually abused, physically abused, and nonabused children. Child Abuse Negl 13:403–408, 1989

Deblinger E, Lippmann J, Steer R: Sexually abused children suffering posttraumatic stress symptoms: initial treatment outcome findings. Child Maltreatment l(4):310–321, 1996

Dykman RA, McPherson B, Ackerman PT, et al: Internalizing and externalizing characteristics of sexually and/or physically abused children. Integrative Physiological and Behavioral Science 32(1):62–74, 1997

Endicott J, Spitzer RL, Fleiss JL, et al: The Global Assessment Scale: a procedure for measuring overall severity of psychiatric disturbance. Arch Gen Psychiatry 33:766-771, 1976

Everson MD, Hunter WM, Runyon DK, etal: Maternal support following disclosure of incest. Am J Orthopsychiatry 59:197–207, 1989

Famularo R, Kinscherff R, Fenton T: Psychiatric diagnoses of maltreated children: preliminary findings. J Am Acad Child Adolesc Psychiatry 31(5):863–867, 1992

Famularo R, Fenton T, Kinscherff R, et al: Maternal and child posttraumatic stress disorder in cases of child maltreatment. Child Abuse Negl 18:27–36, 1994

Field T, Seligman S, Scafidi F, et al: Alleviating posttraumatic stress in children following Hurricane Andrew. Journal of Applied Developmental Psychology 17:37–50, 1996

Finkelhor D, Browne A: The traumatic impact of child sexual abuse: a conceptualization. Am J Orthopsychiatry 55(4):530–541, 1985

Foa EB, Meadows EA: Psychosocial treatment for posttraumatic stress disorder: a critical review. Annu Rev Psychol 48:449–480, 1997

Fonagy P: Evaluating the effectiveness of interventions in child psychiatry. Can J Psychiatry 42:584–594, 1997

Galante R, Foa D: An epidemiological study of psychic trauma and treatment effectiveness for children after a natural disaster. J Am Acad Child Psychiatry 25(3):357–363, 1986

Garrison C, Bryant E, Addy C, et al: Posttraumatic stress disorder in adolescents after Hurricane Andrew. J Am Acad Child Adolesc Psychiatry 34(9):1193–1201, 1995

Giaconia RM, Reinherz HZ, Silverman AB, et al: Traumas and posttraumatic stress disorder in a community population of older adolescents. J Am Acad Child Adolesc Psychiatry 34(10):1369–1380, 1995

Goenjian AK, Karayan I, Pynoos RS, et al: Outcome of psychotherapy among early adolescents after trauma. Am J Psychiatry 154(4):536–542, 1997

Green B, Korol M, Grace M, et al: Children and disaster: age, gender and parental effects on PTSD symptoms. J Am Acad Child Adolesc Psychiatry 30(6):945–951, 1991

Gurwitch RH, Sullivan MA, Long PJ: The impact of trauma and disaster on young children. Child Adolesc Psychiatr Clin N Am 7(1):19–32, 1998

Hamada RS, Kameoka V, Yanagida E: The Kauai Recovery Inventory: Screening for Posttraumatic Stress Symptoms in Children. Article presented at the Annual Meeting of the International Society for Traumatic Stress Studies. San Francisco, CA, November 9–14, 1996

Handford H, Dickerson, Mayes S, et al: Child and parent reaction to the Three Mile Island nuclear accident. J Am Acad Child Adolesc Psychiatry 25:346–356, 1986

Horowitz K, Weine S, Jekel J: PTSD symptoms in urban adolescent girls: compounded community trauma. J Am Acad Child Adolesc Psychiatry 34(10):1353–1361, 1995

Horowitz MJ, Wilner N, Alvarez W: Impact of events scale: a measure of subjective stress. Psychosom Med 41:209–218, 1979

Kazdin AE: Psychotherapy for children and adolescents: current progress and future directions. Am Psychol 48(6):644–657, 1993

Kazdin AE: A model for developing effective treatments: progression and interplay of theory, research, and practice. J Clin Child Psychol 26(2):114–129, 1997

Kazdin AE, Weisz JR: Identifying and developing empirically supported child and adolescent therapy outcome research. J Consult Clin Psychol 66(1):19–36, 1998

Kendall-Tackett KA, Williams LM, Finkelhor D: Impact of sexual abuse on children: a review and synthesis of recent empirical studies. Psychol Bull 113(1):164–180, 1993

Kilpatrick KL, Litt M, Williams LM: Posttraumatic stress disorder in child witnesses to domestic violence. Am J Orthopsychiatry 67(4):639–644, 1997

Kinzie J, Sack W, Angell R, et al: The psychiatric effects of massive trauma on Cambodian children. J Am Acad Child Psychiatry 25(3):370–376, 1986

Kiser LJ, Ackerman BJ, Brown E, et al: Post-traumatic stress disorder in young children: a reaction to purported sexual abuse. J Am Acad Child Adolesc Psychiatry 27(5):645–649, 1988

Knight GP, Kagan S, Buriel R: Perceived parental practices and prosocial development. J Genet Psychol 141:57–65, 1982

Kolko DJ: Individual cognitive behavioral treatment and family therapy for physically abused children and their offending parents: a comparison of clinical outcomes. Child Maltreatment l(4):322–342, 1996

LaGreca A, Silverman W, Vernberg E, et al: Symptoms of posttraumatic stress in children after Hurricane Andrew: a prospective study. J Consult Clin Psychol 64(4):712–723, 1996

Livingston R, Lawson L, Jones J: Predictors of self-reported psychopathology in children abused repeatedly by a parent. J Am Acad Child Adolesc Psychiatry 32(5):948–953, 1993

Malmquist CP: Children who witness parental murder: posttraumatic aspects. J Am Acad Child Adolesc Psychiatry 25(3):320–325, 1986

March JS, Parker, JD, Sullivan KA, et al: The Multidimensional Anxiety Scale for Children (MASC): factor structure, reliability, and validity. J Am Acad Child Adolesc Psychiatry 36(4):554–565, 1997

March J, Amaya-Jackson L, Murray M, et al: Cognitive-behavioral psychotherapy for children and adolescents with posttraumatic stress disorder after a single-incident stressor. J Am Acad Child Adolesc Psychiatry 37(6):585–593, 1998

McGain B, McKinzey RK: The efficacy of group treatment in sexually abused girls. Child Abuse Negl 19(9):1157–1169, 1995

McLeer SV, Deblinger E, Henry D, et al: Sexual abused children at high risk for posttraumatic disorder. J Am Acad Child Adolesc Psychiatry 31(5):865–879, 1992

McLeer SV, Callaghan M, Henry D, et al: Psychiatric disorders in sexually abused children. J Am Acad Child Adolesc Psychiatry 33(3):313–319, 1994

Nader K, Pynoos R, Fairbanks L, et al: Children's PTSD reactions one year after a sniper attack at their school. Am J Psychiatry 147:1526–1530, 1990

Nader K, Blake D, Kriegler J, et al: Clinician Administered PTSD Scale for Children (CAPS-C): Current Lifetime Diagnosis Version and Instruction Manual. Los Angeles, CA, UCLA Neuropsychiatric Institute and National Center for PTSD, 1994

Nowicki S, Strickland BR: A locus of control scale for children. Journal of Consulting Psychology 40:148–154, 1973

Ollendick TH, Yule W, Ollier K: Fears in British children and their relationship to manifest anxiety and depression. J Child Psychol Psychiatry 32:321–331, 1991

Pelcovitz D, Kaplan S, Goldenberg B, et al: Posttraumatic stress disorder in physically abused adolescents. J Am Acad Child Adolesc Psychiatry 33(3):305–312, 1994

Pelcovitz D, Libov B, Mandel F, et al: Posttraumatic stress disorder and family functioning in adolescent cancer. J Trauma Stress 11(2):205–221, 1998

Peterson L, Brown D: Integrating child injury and abuse-neglect research: common histories, etiologies, and solutions. Psychol Bull 116(2):293–315, 1994

Poe-Yamagata E: Number of children reported to protective service agencies, 1980–1996. Adapted from Sickmund M, Snyder H, Poe-Yamagata E: Juvenile Offenders and Victims: 1997 Update on Violence. Washington, DC, U.S. Department of Justice, Office of Justice Programs, Office of Juvenile Justice and Delinquency Prevention, 1997

Pynoos R, Frederick C, Nader K, et al: Life threat and posttraumatic stress in school-age children. Arch Gen Psychiatry 44:1057–1063, 1987

Reynolds CR, Richmond BO: What I think and feel: a revised measure of children's manifest anxiety. J Abnorm Child Psychol 271–280, 1978

Reynolds CR, Richmond BO: Revised Children's Manifest Anxiety Scale Manual. Los Angeles, CA, Western Psychological Services, 1985

Schwarz E, Kowalski J: Posttraumatic stress disorder after a school shooting: effects of symptom threshold selection and diagnosis by DSM-III, DSM-III-R or proposed DSM-IV. Am J Psychiatry 148:592–597, 1991

Shaffer D, Gould MS, Brasic J, et al: A Children's Global Assessment Scale (CGAS). Arch Gen Psychiatry 40:1228–1231, 1983

Shannon M, Lonigan C, Finch A, et al: Children exposed to disaster, I: epidemiology of posttraumatic symptoms and symptom profile. J Am Acad Child Adolesc Psychiatry 33(1):80–93, 1994

Shaw J, Applegate B, Tanner S, et al: Psychological effects of Hurricane Andrew on an elementary school population. J Am Acad Child Adolesc Psychiatry 34(9): 1185–1192, 1995

Spielberger C: Preliminary Test Manual for the State-Trait Anxiety Inventory for Children. Palo Alto, CA, Consulting Psychologists Press, 1973

Spielberger CD, Johnson EH, Russell SF, et al: The experience and expression of anger: construction and validatiion of an anger expression scale, in Anger and Hostility in Cardiovascular and Behavioral Disorders. Edited by Chesney MA, Rosenman RH. New York, Hemisphere/McGraw Hill, 1985, pp 5–30.

Solomon SD, Gerrity ET, Muff AM, et al: Efficacy of treatments for posttraumatic stress disorder. JAMA 268(5):633–638, 1992

Stallard P, Velleman R, Baldwin S, et al: Prospective study of posttraumatic stress disorder in children involved in road traffic accidents. BMJ 317:1691–1693, 1998

Stuber ML, Nader K, Yasuda P, et al: Stress responses after pediatric bone marrow transplantation: preliminary results of a prospective longitudinal study. J Am Acad Child Adolesc Psychiatry 30(6):952–957, 1991

Sullivan PM, Scanlan JM, Bookhouser PE, et al: The effects of psychotherapy on behavior problems of sexually abused deaf children. Child Abuse Negl 16:297–397, 1992

Terr LC: Psychic trauma in children: observations following the Chowchilla school bus kidnapping. Am J Psychiatry 138(1):14–19, 1981

Tonkins SAM, Lambert MJ: A treatment outcome study of bereavement groups for children. Child and Adolescent Social Work Journal 13(1):3–21, 1996

Verleur D, Hughes RE, de Rios DM: Enhancement of self-esteem among female adolescent incest victims: a controlled comparison. Adolescence 21(84):843–854, 1986

Wagar JM, Rodway MR: An evaluation of a group treatment approach for children who have witnessed wife abuse. Journal of Family Violence 10(3):295–306, 1995

Wolf VV, Gentile C, Michienzi T, et al: The Children's Impact of Traumatic Events Scale: a measure of post-sexual abuse PTSD symptoms. Behavioral Assessment 13:359–383, 1991

Yule W: Posttraumatic stress disorder in child survivors of shipping disasters: the sinking of the "Jupiter." Psychother Psychosom 57:200–205, 1992

6

Assessment and Treatment of Complex PTSD

Bessel A. van der Kolk, M.D.

Trauma as an etiologic agent in the genesis of psychopathology was largely ignored from the end of the second world war until about 40 years later. During that time, trauma-based psychiatric problems were generally trivialized, as exemplified by the following quote about the impact of childhood sexual abuse in the leading textbook of psychiatry in 1972:

> [Incest is thought to occur] in approximately 1 out of 1.1 million women. There is little agreement about the role of father-daughter incest as a source of serious subsequent psychopathology. The father-daughter liaison satisfies instinctual drives in a setting where mutual alliance with an omnipotent adult condones the transgression.... The act offers an opportunity to test in reality an infantile fantasy whose consequences are found to be gratifying and pleasurable.... The ego's capacity for sublimation is favored by the pleasure afforded by incest.... Such incestuous activity diminishes the subject's chance of psychosis and allows for a better adjustment to the external world.
>
> There is often found little deleterious influence on the subsequent

I wish to acknowledge the helpful comments and suggestions on this chapter by Drs. Janina Fisher, Debbie Korn, Onno van der Hart, Pat Ogden, Joseph Spinazzola, and Peter Levine.

personality of the incestuous daughter.... One study found that the vast majority of them were none the worse for the experience. (Freedman et al. 1972)

After the Vietnam War, the psychopathological effects of traumatization that were seen in hundreds of thousands of Vietnam veterans resulted in the diagnosis of posttraumatic stress disorder (PTSD) being created for inclusion in DSM-III (American Psychiatric Association 1980).

However, over the years it has become clear that in clinical settings the majority of traumatized persons seeking treatment have a variety of psychological problems that are not included in the diagnosis of PTSD. These include depression and self-hatred; dissociation and depersonalization; aggressive behavior against self and others; problems with intimacy; and impairment in the capacity to experience pleasure and satisfaction. Many of these problems that are not included under the rubric of PTSD are classified as comorbid conditions rather than being recognized as part of a spectrum of treatment-resistant, trauma-related problems. These problems seem to occur as a function of the developmental level at which the trauma occurred, the relationship between the victim and the agent responsible for the trauma, the duration of the traumatic experiences, and the availability of social support

A DSM-IV Field Trial (van der Kolk et al. 1996a, 1996b, 1996c) demonstrated that the distinguishing factor between a group of individuals with PTSD who sought treatment and another group with PTSD who did not seek treatment was not the prevalence of PTSD symptoms themselves but the presence of depression; outbursts of anger; self-destructive behavior; and feelings of shame, self-blame, and distrust. The notion that the majority of people who seek treatment for trauma-related problems have histories of multiple traumas is exemplified in Table 6–1, which shows the trauma histories of 70 individuals who consecutively sought treatment in our trauma center outpatient clinic during April and May 1999.

Although these trauma center patients had a mean PTSD score of 73 (equivalent to the same score on the Clinician-Administered PTSD Scale), they had a variety of other psychological problems, which in most cases were the chief presenting complaints: 77% showed significant dysregulation of affects and impulses, including aggression against self and others; 84% reported depersonalization and other dissociative symptoms; 75% had chronic feelings of shame, self-blame, and feeling permanently damaged; 83% complained of being unable to negotiate satisfactory relationships with others; and 73% said they had lost previously sustaining beliefs. Our patients reported that these problems, rather than the intrusive recollections characteristic of PTSD, made their lives unbearable.

TABLE 6–1. Percentage of different trauma types reported by 70 patients consecutively admitted to a trauma center

Trauma type	Age at occurrence				Lifetime
	0–6	7–12	13–18	19+	
Separation and loss	47.1	61.4	81.4	84.3	98.6
Neglect	58.2	71.4	81.1	80.0	91.4
Physical abuse	41.4	54.3	55.7	50.0	80.0
Sexual abuse	25.7	41.4	41.4	44.3	74.3
Emotional abuse	51.4	77.1	85.7	82.9	85.7
Other traumas	50.0	55.7	65.7	82.9	91.4
Witnessing violence	54.3	71.4	78.6	70.0	87.1
Familial substance abuse	40.0	50.0	67.1	65.7	75.7

PTSD has become a common diagnosis for psychiatric inpatients. For example, an examination of the records of the 384,000 Medicaid recipients in Massachusetts in 1997–98 (Macy 1999) revealed that PTSD and depression were the most common psychiatric diagnoses. However, patients with a PTSD diagnosis spent 10 times as much time in the hospital than patients with the diagnosis of depression only. It is inconceivable that the 22,800 Medicaid recipients in Massachusetts who were hospitalized and diagnosed with PTSD between 1997 and 1998 were admitted after a one-time traumatic incident, such as a rape or motor vehicle accident. Most likely, they experienced a complex constellation of symptoms, like those of the patients at the trauma center, which led to their requiring hospitalization.

However, because the long-term psychiatric impact of chronic, multiple traumas is classified under the same rubric (PTSD) as would be the sequelae of a one-time incident, there is no formal way of describing how convoluted the psychiatric presentations of these patients are and how complex their treatment is. In Macy's Medicaid sample, a small group of 1,200 patients with dissociative identity disorder—a diagnosis associated with severe and prolonged interpersonal childhood trauma—had by far the highest utilization rate of any psychiatric diagnosis in Massachusetts during the years 1997 and 1998. Yet there currently is not a single funded research program studying the phenomenology and treatment of this disorder in the United States.

PTSD as a Diagnostic Construct

PTSD as a diagnosis was constructed in response to a social demand to delineate a syndrome that described the psychological suffering experienced by many Vietnam combat veterans at a time when the United States was coping with millions of soldiers who had just returned from the war. Before the creation of the diagnosis of PTSD, other posttraumatic syndromes had been proposed, such as rape trauma syndrome (Burgess and Holstrom 1974) and battered woman syndrome (Walker 1977/1978). Those syndromes highlighted the effects of those assaults on the victims' sense of safety, trust, and self-worth and on their continued sense of terror. Guided by Kardiner's (1941) description of the "traumatic neuroses of war" and Horowitz's (1974) biphasic stress response syndrome, the DSM-III definition of PTSD highlighted the physiologic alterations that follow traumatization and the coexisting traumatic intrusions and emotional numbing and avoidance.

Although numerous studies have demonstrated that the diagnostic construct of PTSD describes essential elements of the suffering caused by such traumas as rape, torture, child abuse, and motor vehicle accidents, no large-factor analysis has been conducted across a variety of trauma populations to test whether the diagnostic criteria for PTSD uniquely capture the psychological damage that occurs in response to psychologically overwhelming experiences. The PTSD Field Trial failed to measure other Axis I or Axis II disorders in its sample of 528 traumatized individuals. Therefore, the design of the DSM-IV field trial was unable to demonstrate that the criteria delineated in the diagnosis of PTSD capture the most essential elements of human suffering that occurs in the wake of trauma. However, the field trial did provide some information about how trauma at different ages contributes to the genesis of a complex constellation of symptoms that came to be called disorders of extreme stress not otherwise specified, or complex PTSD.

Childhood Trauma and Complex PTSD

At our urban outpatient clinic, which specializes in the treatment of traumatized children and adults, most patients who seek treatment have histories of chronic emotional, physical, and sexual abuse. This is not surprising, as childhood trauma is very common in our society and its effects are well documented to persist over time. Each year over 3 million children are reported for abuse and/or neglect in the United States (Wang and Daro 1997). Only about a third of abused and neglected children in clinical settings meet diagnostic criteria for PTSD. For example, in one study of 364 abused children (Ackerman et al. 1998) (Table 6–2), the most common diagnoses in order of frequency were separation anxiety disorder, oppositional defiant disorder, phobic disorders, PTSD, and attention-deficit/hyperactivity disorder. Although abused and neglected children may receive a variety of psychiatric labels, none of these diagnoses capture the profound developmental disturbances nor the traumatic origins of the particular clinical presentations. Regardless of the diagnoses they receive, these children tend to be characterized by pervasive problems with attachment, attention, and managing physiological arousal.

There is little indication that children "outgrow" these early problems: people with histories of early abuse and neglect have repeatedly been found to have profound and pervasive psychiatric problems. Their problems with negotiating satisfying interpersonal relationships seem to play a particularly significant role in preventing them from leading satisfying lives; being able to engage in competent social relationships has been shown to be an important prognostic factor in the capacity to recover from traumatic experiences (e.g., Ford et al. 1997; van der Kolk et al. 1991).

Childhood abuse and neglect have been shown to profoundly impair the capacity for self-regulation (Cicchetti and Toth 1995; Kendall-Tackett

TABLE 6–2. Abuse groups

Diagnosis	Total (%)	Sexual (N=127)		Physical (N=43)		Both (N=34)		Control[a] (%)
		Boys (%)	Girls (%)	Boys (%)	Girls (%)	Boys (%)	Girls (%)	
ADHD	29	40	22	36	10	67	26	3–5
Oppositional defiant disorder	36	46	22	56	20	64	47	6.5
Conduct disorder	21	44	11	21	10	67	21	3.9
Major depression	13	12	11	12	20	8	32	0.4–8.3
Bipolar disorders	9	4	9	9	20	0	21	1
Dysthymia	19	16	13	24	20	17	42	
Separation anxiety/overanxious	59	44	58	48	100	59	79	2.9–4.6
Phobic	36	44	36	24	30	25	58	2.4–9.2
Obsessive-compulsive disorder	14	0	14	18	20	8	27	0.5
PTSD	34	20	35	18	50	58	53	>6

Note: Of subjects included, 62% were outpatients, 25% were inpatients, and 13% were referred from local agencies.
ADHD=attention-deficit/hyperactivity disorder; PTSD=posttraumatic stress disorder.
[a]Based on various studies.
Source: Ackerman et al. 1998.

et al. 1993; Rodriguez et al. 1997; Westen et al. 1990a, 1990b). Chronic affect dysregulation, in turn, is associated with substance use (Chilcoat and Breslau 1998), chronic anxiety and depression (Beitchman et al. 1992; Felitti et al. 1998; Polusny and Follette 1995), and increased use of medical and mental health services (Drossman et al. 1990; Felitti et al. 1998; Golding et al. 1988; Moeller et al. 1993; Rapkin et al. 1990).

In clinical settings, pervasive problems with self-regulation are most readily evident in the patients experiencing even minor objective stressors as overwhelming, and their managing the resulting distress with self-destructive behaviors, such as self-injury, substance use, eating disorders, and suicide attempts (Felitti et al. 1998; Putnam 1999; van der Kolk et al. 1991). Loss of self-regulation may be expressed on other levels as well: as a loss of ability to focus on relevant stimuli, as attentional problems, and as an inability to inhibit action when aroused. Such problems with attention and stimulus discrimination may account for the high comorbidity between PTSD and attention-deficit/hyperactivity disorder in traumatized children, such as sexually abused girls (Putnam 1997).

Having a history of childhood abuse and neglect predisposes individuals to develop PTSD in response to subsequent traumatic stressors (Bremner et al. 1993; Widom 1999). Childhood trauma is also associated with the development of borderline personality disorder (e.g., Herman et al. 1989; Ogata et al. 1990), somatization disorder (e.g., Saxe et al. 1994), dissociative disorders (e.g., Kluft 1991; Putnam 1989; Ross et al. 1989, 1991; Saxe et al. 1993), and eating disorders (DeGroot et al. 1992; Herzog et al. 1993; McFarlane et al. 1988).

In summary, abused and neglected children, and many adults with histories of abuse and neglect, tend to have 1) a lack of a predictable sense of self, with a poor sense of separateness, and a disturbed body image; 2) poorly modulated affect and impulse control, including aggression against self and others; and 3) uncertainty about the reliability and predictability of others. This accounts for the distrust, suspiciousness, problems with intimacy, and social isolation seen in many individuals with these histories. Cole and Putnam (1992) proposed that people's core sense of self is defined to a substantial degree by their capacity to regulate internal states and by how well they can predict and regulate their responses to stress. Thus, it is not surprising that the first order of therapy should focus on establishing a capacity for affect regulation.

Trauma and Personality Development

For children, the principal source of information about who they are is the quality of their relationships with their parents. Therefore, it is not surprising that abused and neglected children are faced with enormous challenges to construct meaningful lives and safe interpersonal relationships. The combination of a lack of adequate self-regulatory processes; chronic dissociation; physical problems without a clear medical cause; and exposure to caregivers who are cruel, inconsistent, exploitive, unresponsive, or violent is likely to have a profound impact on the sense of who one is. It is also likely to lead to disturbances of body image; a view of oneself as helpless, damaged, and ineffective; and difficulties with trust, intimacy, and self-assertion (Cole and Putnam 1992; Herman 1992; van der Kolk 1987; van der Kolk and Fisler 1995).

To a considerable degree, the effects of traumatic exposure depend the developmental level of the individual when the trauma occurs (Pynoos et al. 1996). However, it has been repeatedly noted that previously well-functioning traumatized adults often have a significant decline in their overall functioning as well. Such "posttraumatic decline" following adult trauma was already well documented in the literature of the Second World War (e.g., Archibald and Tuddenham 1965). Kardiner (1941, p. 82) noted that, once traumatized, "the subject acts as if the original traumatic situation were still in existence and engages in protective devices which failed on the original occasion." This means in effect that "his conception of the outer world and his conception of himself have been permanently altered." (p. 249).

Trauma-based cognitive schemes come to organize traumatized individuals' views of themselves and their surroundings. Often, there are coexisting parallel schemes, which are activated in a state-dependent manner: high levels of competence and interpersonal sensitivity can exist side by side with self-hatred, lack of self-care, and interpersonal cruelty (Crittenden 1988). Many people who were traumatized in their own families have great difficulty taking care of their own basic needs (e.g., hygiene, rest, and protection), even as they may be exquisitely responsive to other people's needs. Many repeat their family patterns in interpersonal relationships, in which they may alternate between being victim or persecutor, often justifying their behavior by their feelings of betrayal and helplessness. The use of projective identification—attributing to others one's own most despised attributes, and acting on the basis of that projection without being able to acknowledge the existence of those characteristics in oneself—has been well described by Kernberg (1975).

Disorders of Extreme Stress (DESNOS)

In preparation for a possible revision of the definition of PTSD in DSM-IV, some members of the PTSD task force delineated a syndrome of psychological problems that have been shown to be frequently associated with histories of prolonged and severe interpersonal abuse. This conglomeration of symptoms has been called complex PTSD, or disorders of extreme stress not otherwise specified (DESNOS) (Herman 1992; van der Kolk et al. 1996c). The diagnosis consisted of six different problems that research had shown to be associated with early interpersonal trauma: 1) alterations in the regulation of affective impulses, including difficulty with modulation of anger and being self-destructive; 2) alterations in attention and consciousness leading to amnesias and dissociative episodes and depersonalizations; 3) alterations in self-perception, such as a chronic sense of guilt and responsibility or chronically feeling ashamed; 4) alterations in relationship to others, such as not being able to trust or not being able to feel intimate with people; 5) somatization the problem of feeling symptoms on a somatic level for which no medical explanations can be found; and 6) alterations in systems of meaning (see Table 6–3).

TABLE 6–3. Symptoms of disorders of extreme stress (DESNOS) or complex PTSD

1. Impairment of affect regulation
2. Chronic destructive behavior
    Self-mutilation
    Eating disorders
    Drug abuse, etc.
3. Amnesia and dissociation
4. Somatization
5. Alterations in relationship to self
6. Distorted relations with others
7. Loss of sustaining beliefs

The DSM-IV Field Trial of PTSD found that DESNOS had a high construct validity (Pelcovitz et al. 1997). The earlier the onset of the trauma, and the longer the duration, the more likely people were to experience high degrees of all the symptoms that make up the DESNOS diagnosis (Figure 6–1). The DESNOS construct has been assessed in community (Roth et al. 1997; van der Kolk et al. 1996c) and in specialized inpatient (Ford 1999; Ford and Kidd 1998) and outpatient mental health settings (Roth et al. 1997; van der Kolk et al. 1996c). These studies showed that interpersonal trauma, especially childhood abuse, predicts a higher risk for the development of DESNOS than do accidents and disasters (Roth et al. 1997).

Ford and Kidd (1998) found that meeting diagnostic criteria for

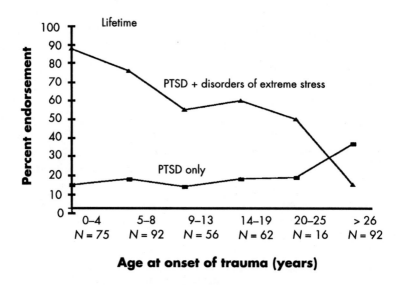

FIGURE 6–1. Percentage endorsement of all categories of disorders of extreme stress not otherwise specified (DESNOS) by age at onset of trauma, as reported in the DSM-IV Field Trial of posttraumatic stress disorder (PTSD).

DESNOS, and not a history of early developmental trauma per se, distinguished therapeutic outcome. Ford (1999) found that despite substantial overlap between PTSD and DESNOS, the two conditions had substantially different symptomatic and functional impairment features. In contrast with the DSM-IV Field Trial, which found a 92% comorbidity between DESNOS and PTSD, Ford and Kidd (1998) found that DESNOS could occur in the absence of PTSD and that DESNOS was associated with particularly severe self-reported intrusive reexperiencing symptomatology, over and above that attributable to PTSD.

Why Do We Need DESNOS?

PTSD patients with DESNOS frequently do not respond to conventional PTSD treatment and may in fact be harmed by it (Ford 1999). McDonagh-Coyle et al. (1999) conducted a randomized, controlled trial of combined prolonged exposure and cognitive restructuring (PE/CR) versus "present-centered therapy" (PCT) that specifically did not involve either prolonged exposure or cognitive restructuring. Attrition was high in PE/CR (30%) but low in PCT (10%). PCT was equally effective in reducing PTSD and psychiatric symptoms and in making clinically significant reductions in research-diagnosed PTSD. These results suggest that some adults who were abused and neglected as children and who currently meet diagnostic criteria for PTSD may react adversely to PE/CR, and that effective treatment may need to focus on self-regulatory deficits rather than on PE/CR.

The literature on treatment failures with prolonged exposure suggests that patients who have the DESNOS constellation of symptoms are the least responsive to that treatment and that it may in fact aggravate their condition. Subjects with the poorest outcomes in PE/CR are characterized by high initial levels of anger (Foa et al. 1995); memories during reliving of the trauma reflecting "mental defeat" or the absence of mental planning (Ehlers et al. 1998); a feeling of alienation or being permanently damaged by the trauma (Ehlers et al. 1998); and an inability to develop a nonfragmentary, coherent narrative recounting of trauma experiences during reliving of the trauma in treatment (Foa et al. 1997). The parallel between these features and DESNOS is quite striking. Moreover, a recent study showed that individuals with DESNOS tended to have deficits in developmentally based self-regulatory capacities and responded poorly to treatment in a multimodal milieu PTSD treatment program (Ford and Kidd 1998).

Assessment of Traumatized Patients

Although PTSD has become the central organizing diagnosis for traumatized patients, it does not take into account the complexity of adaptation to trauma, nor does a patient's PTSD score inform clinicians about such relevant issues as functional impairment, developmental aspects of the trauma, what resources the patient has available to deal with his or her PTSD symptoms, and how different traumatizing life events have coalesced to give rise to the current clinical picture.

To formulate a rational treatment plan it is critical to be aware of the patient's premorbid history and available coping resources. To this end our trauma center has developed a computerized Traumatic Antecedents Questionnaire (TAQ), which gathers information about the patients' resources (having particular competencies and feeling safe with potentially protective people) during different stages of development: ages 0–6, 7–12, 13–18, and adulthood. In addition to measuring resources, it also assesses a variety of potentially traumatizing events over all developmental periods, including neglect, separations from significant others, secrets, emotional abuse, physical abuse, sexual abuse, witnessing, other traumas, and exposure to alcohol and drugs. A computer printout allows the clinician to gain a rapid overview both of the history of resources and of potentially traumatizing life events (see Figure 6–2 for a sample printout).

Name:
I.D.: 2223fabs
Date: 10/23/9_

Traumatic Antecedents Questionnaire

	Young child (0–6)	School age (7–12)	Adolescence (13–18)	Adulthood	Total
Resources					
Competence	3.0	3.0	2.0	2.5	10.5
Safety	3.0	2.0	0.0	0.0	5.0
Trauma and neglect					
Neglect	0.0	0.0	0.0	NA	0.0
Separation	0.0	3.0	3.0	3.0	9.0
Secrets	2.0	0.0	2.0	0.0	4.0
Emotional abuse	0.0	2.0	0.0	3.0	9.0
Physical abuse	0.0	0.0	3.0	3.0	6.0
Sexual abuse	0.0	0.0	0.0	3.0	0.0
Witnessing	3.0	0.0	2.0	3.0	8.0
Other traumas	0.0	0.0	2.0	3.0	5.0
Alcohol and drugs	3.0	0.0	2.0	3.0	8.0

Key: 0=Not at all, never, a little bit, or rarely; numbers between 2.0 and 3.0 are averages of endorsed items meaning moderately, somewhat (2.0) to often, very much (3.0)

FIGURE 6–2. Sample printout of Traumatic Antecedents Questionnaire (TAQ). This is the TAQ profile of a 29-year-old chronically battered woman, presenting in great distress. She had a violent alcoholic father, who left the family when the patient was 6 years old. In adolescence she engaged in alcohol and drug abuse and married a violent alcoholic man. Her memory of early safety and life-long sense of competence are expected to positively affect her long-term prognosis.

Patients also fill out a computerized PTSD rating scale and the computerized Structured Interview for Disorders of Extreme Stress (Pelcovitz et al. 1997), which measures the items enumerated in DESNOS: 1) alteration in regulation of affect and impulses; 2) alterations in attention of consciousness; 3) alterations in self-perceptions; 4) alterations in relationship to others; 5) somatization; and 6) alterations in belief systems (see Figure 6–3 for a sample printout). Having thus obtained a developmental history of both coping resources and trauma-related symptomatology allows clinicians to prioritize the appropriate treatment interventions. (Copies of these assessment instruments can be obtained by visiting our web site at http://www.traumacenter.org.)

The most important issue we evaluate is the capacity of our patients to

Name
ID: 2223FABS
Date: 10/23/9_

	Present	Current severity
I. Alteration in regulation of affect and impulses		? 5
Ia) Affect regulation:	Yes	3.0
Ib) Modulation of anger:	Yes	2.0
Ic) Self-destructive:	Yes	0.0
Id) Suicidal preoccupation:	Yes	3.0
Ie) Difficulty modulating sexual involvement preoccupation:	Yes	0.0
If Excessive risk taking:	No	0.0
II. Alterations in attention or consciousness	Yes	1.5
IIa) Amnesia	Yes	0.0
IIb) Transient dissociative episodes and depersonalization	Yes	2.0
III. Alteration in Self-Perception		2.0
IIIa) Ineffectiveness:	Yes	3.0
IIIb) Permanent damage:	Yes	2.0
IIIc) Guilt and responsibility:	No	0.0
IIId) Shame:	Yes	3.0
IIIe) Nobody can understand:	Yes	2.0
IIIf) Minimizing:	No	0.0
IV. Alterations in relationships with others		1.5
IVa) Inability to trust:	Yes	3.0
IVb) Revictimization:	No	0.0
IVc) Victimizing others:	No	0.0
V. Somatization	Yes	0.6
Va) Digestive system:	Yes	0.6
Vb) Chronic pain:	Yes	3.0
Vc) Cardiopulmonary symptoms:	Yes	0.0
Vd) Conversion symptoms:	Yes	0.0
Ve) Sexual symptoms	No	0.0
VI. Alterations in systems of meaning		3.0
VIa) Foreshortened future:	Yes	3.0
VIb) Loss of previously sustained beliefs	No	3.0

FIGURE 6–3. Sample scoring report, Structured Interview for Disorders of Extreme Stress.

modulate their affective arousal: whether they are able to be emotionally upset without hurting themselves, becoming aggressive, or dissociating. As long as they cannot do this, addressing the trauma is likely to lead to negative therapeutic outcomes. Similarly, as long as they dissociate when they feel upset they will be unable to take charge of their lives and will be unable to "process" traumatic experiences. Hence, a substantial part of the treatment of our chronically traumatized patients consists of stabilization and the development of resources to cope with both the sequelae of their earlier trauma and the challenges of day-to-day life.

Treatment Approaches to Chronically Traumatized Individuals

In contrast to traumas such as motor vehicle accidents and torture, childhood abuse occurs as a part of ordinary everyday life. Therefore, for people who have been abused as children, seemingly innocuous experiences, ostensibly harmless sounds, the way light comes into a window, particular smells, and physical sensations may become triggers of extreme emotional distress. When triggered by traumatic reminders the past becomes the present.

Therapists who treat chronically traumatized patients need to develop a keen appreciation of how trauma is reenacted. They need to help patients accurately evaluate and process their current situations and their physical and emotional responses to the present and avoid participating in any reenactment of patients' past dramas. Because interpersonal trauma tends to occur in contexts in which the rules are unclear, under circumstances that are secret, and in conditions where issues of responsibility are often murky, patients will be exquisitely sensitive to issues of rules, boundaries, contracts, and mutual responsibilities (Herman 1992; Kluft 1992). They are prone to misinterpret minor frustrations as a return of past insults. Rather than understanding uncomfortable sensations as memories that have been triggered by some current event, they act as if only restorative action in the present could alter the way they feel. Inexperienced therapists often take on the challenge to ameliorate the past by trying to provide restorative experiences in the present. This usually leads to a repetition, rather than a resolution, of the trauma.

Because they tend to have physiologic reactions to triggers of traumatic reminders, these patients are prone to experience slight irritations as emergencies and blame people in their surroundings for the way they feel. Hence these patients, while numbing and dissociating in the face of real violations, often experience minor frustrations within the therapeutic relationship itself as violations. As a consequence, these patients are most at risk of being abused by their therapists and by those in the medical profession in general and, reciprocally, to be experienced by those in the medical profession as abusive, ungrateful, and manipulative.

Phase-Oriented Treatment

All treatment of traumatized individuals needs to be paced according to the degree of involuntary intrusion of the trauma and the individual's capacities to deal with intense affects, while understanding and respecting the various psychic defenses that are utilized to deal with the memories of traumatic material. For more than a century, clinicians have advocated the application of phase-oriented treatment that includes 1) establishing a diagnosis, including prioritizing the range of problems experienced by the individual, and 2) designing a realistic phase-oriented treatment plan, consisting of

- Stabilization, including identification of feelings by verbalizing somatic states.
- Deconditioning of traumatic memories and responses.
- Integration of traumatic personal schemes.
- Reestablishing secure social connections and interpersonal efficacy.
- Accumulating restitutive emotional experiences. (Herman 1992; van der Kolk et al. 1996c).

In the treatment of single-incident trauma, it is often possible to move quickly from one phase to the next; in cases of complex chronic interpersonal abuse, clinicians often need to refocus on stabilization (e.g., Briere 1996; Brown and Fromm 1986; Chu 1998; Courtois 1991; Herman 1992; Janet 1919/1925; van der Kolk et al. 1996). Table 6–4 summarizes what appears to be the consensus by experts in this area about the appropriate stage-oriented treatment approach to patients with complex PTSD (van der Kolk et al. 1996c).

Trauma and the Body

The foundation of self-awareness and self-regulation rests on understanding the nuances and meaning of one's of physical sensations. The way people feel and the way they interpret the meaning of incoming information depends, to a large degree, on the meaning that they assign to their physical sensations (Schachtel 1947). As people develop they learn how to interpret, manage, and act on internal physical sensations. These can be generated internally (as in hunger, sleep, and the need to urinate or defecate) or by interactions between the self and the surrounding world, as is the perception of fearful, soothing, or pleasurable stimuli. As children mature they gradually learn to interpret their bodily sensations, to attach emotional valence to them, and to take appropriate action. It is thought that care-

TABLE 6–4.   Phase-oriented treatment of complex posttraumatic stress
disorder (disorder of extreme stress not otherwise specified)

Manage symptoms: medications, dialectical behavior therapy, mindfulness
training, stress inoculation training

Create narratives

Realize repetitive patterns

Make connections between internal states and actions:

Aggression

Sex

Eating

Gambling

Cutting

Identify traumatic memory nodes, followed by

Exposure therapy

Eye movement desensitization and reprocessing

Body-oriented work

Learn interpersonal connections: 12 steps, negotiation of sharing responsibility
and intimacy

givers play a critical role in helping to modulate children's physiologic arousal by providing a balance between soothing and stimulation. This "affect attunement" (Stern 1985) between caregivers and infants regulates normal play and exploratory activity. By learning to coordinate physical sensations into a coherent whole, children develop a predictable sense of self. As children mature, they gradually become less vulnerable to overstimulation and learn to tolerate higher levels of excitement. As long as the environment is more or less predictable, children gradually learn how to effectively take care of themselves. When that occurs they have less need for physical proximity of a caregiver to maintain comfort, and they start spending more time playing by themselves and with their peers (Field 1985). Secure children simultaneously learn how to get help when they are distressed. By accumulating a store of effective actions, they learn to predict the most appropriate response to most situations, and, failing that, when to look for outside help to cope.

Cicchetti and Carlson (1989) have shown that traumatized children follow different developmental routes: 80% of them have disorganized attachment patterns. This interferes with their capacity to regulate physiologic states and manifests itself in chronic patterns of hypoarousal and hyperarousal. This is likely to persist throughout the life cycle and will probably make these already traumatized individuals vulnerable to further traumatization. When children become overwhelmed by physiologic arousal and caregivers fail to help them to re-regulate themselves, they fail to acquire the necessary capacity to use physical sensations as guides for effective action. Instead, they tend to become disorganized in response to minor stresses.

Porges et al. (1998) showed that the capacity to modulate arousal is, at least to some extent, genetically based and that some children are much more vulnerable to lack of adequate parental care than others because of greater innate physiologic reactivity. It has long been postulated that difficulty tolerating and interpreting somatic sensations tends to promote the development of alexithymia (Krystal 1978). This inability to evaluate the emotional significance of sensate experience keeps these people from learning from experience and prevents them from engaging in meaningful actions that can provide relief. Their disorganized states are merely experienced as diffuse physical discomfort, emotional distress, lack of energy, or feelings of being dead. Reports of somatic symptoms for which no clear organic pathology can be found is ubiquitous in the psychiatric literature on traumatized children and adults (for a review, see Saxe et al. 1994) and include chronic back and neck pain, fibromyalgias, migraines, digestive problems, spastic colon/irritable bowel, allergies, thyroid and other endocrine disorders, anxiety, depression, chronic fatigue, and some forms of asthma. Together these symptoms may explain some of the remarkable increase in rates of medical morbidity, mortality, and medical service utilization that was documented by Felitti et al. (1998).

When certain bodily signals become harbingers of helplessness and defeat—instead of subtle physical shifts that denote warning, satisfaction, or pleasure—people often learn to avoid feeling them. As a result, these individuals tend to lack nuanced responses to frustrations and go out of control in the face of stress and respond with excessive anger and impulsivity or by becoming depersonalized, "spaced out," or numb. Whatever the behavioral expression, these persons generally are unable to define the precise challenge they are facing. This may contribute not only to their well-documented lack of self-protection and high rates of revictimization (Brownet al. 1998), but also to their remarkable lack of capacity for feeling pleasure and meaning.

To overcome the effects of this physical hyperarousal and numbing, it is critical for traumatized people is to find words to identify bodily sensations and to name emotional states. Knowing what one feels and allowing oneself to experience uncomfortable sensations and emotions is essential in planning how to cope with these sensations and emotions. Freud (1911/1959) postulated that, to function properly, people need to be able to define their needs and to entertain a range of options on how to meet them, without resorting to premature action to make those feelings go away. He called this: "thought as experimental action." Being able to name and tolerate sensations, feelings, and experiences gives people the capacity to "own" what they feel. Being "in touch' with oneself is indispensable for mastery and for having the mental flexibility to contrast and compare and to imagine a range of alternative outcomes (aside from a recurrence of the trauma).

As long as patients vacillate between extremes of underarousal and overarousal, it is difficult to distinguish current frustrations from past trauma, and hence these individuals are prone to react to the present as a return of the past. People need to have the skills to calm themselves down before they are ready to confront their traumatic memories. Without it, exposure is likely to be retraumatizing, because intense affects are likely to overwhelm the patient just as they did at the time of the original trauma. When traumatized individuals feel out of control and unable to modulate their distress, they are vulnerable to resorting to pathological self-soothing behaviors, such as substance abuse, binge eating, self-injury, or clinging to potentially dangerous partners.

Trapped between feeling too much and feeling too little, many traumatized individuals devote their energy to avoiding the uncontrollable sensations associated with pain and helplessness. One way of doing this is by looking for a person, often in the form of a therapist, who can help them do what their early caregivers failed to provide at critical moments: supply them with comfort and safety. Others do this by seeking sensations and experiences that will keep them out of touch by means of engaging in compulsions, addictions, and distractions that keep them from experiencing physical sensations associated with fear and helplessness.

Teaching terrified people to safely experience their sensations and emotions has not been given sufficient attention in mainstream trauma treatment. With the advent of effective medications, such as the selective serotonin reuptake inhibitors (e.g., van der Kolk et al. 1994), medications increasingly have taken the place of teaching people skills to deal with uncomfortable physical sensations. The most natural way that humans beings calm themselves down when feeling distressed and overwhelmed is by holding, hugging, and rocking. This seems to allow them to regain the capacity to overcome excessive arousal and return to feeling intact: capable of tolerating physical experience. This yearning for physical comfort is usually reactivated in relationships in which traumatized people reexamine their experiences with threat and abandonment. In traditional one-on-one therapeutic settings, particularly with patients with histories of physical invasion, adults acting on those longings will tend to activate, rather than heal, the confusion between safety and violation, although helping to feel and tolerate those sensations and fostering relationships in which they can be safely expressed should be a central therapeutic task.

However, there is a long-standing tradition of specific body-oriented treatment techniques—first articulated by Wilhelm Reich (1937), and in modern times expanded to trauma-specific body-oriented work (e.g., Gendlin 1998; Levine and Frederick 1997) and psychodramatic techniques (e.g., Pesso and Crandell 1991)—focusing on experiencing, tolerating, and transforming trauma-related physical sensations. Those traditions are widely practiced outside of academic and medical settings. Unfortunately, at present it is difficult to obtain reimbursement for employing such techniques, and it is impossible to obtain grants to study them.

Symptom Management

Attending to issues of day-to-day safety, self-care, connections with other human beings, and competence is a critical element in the therapy of chronically traumatized individuals. The therapist's job is not just to focus on issues of sorrow, fear, and pain and to actively work on gaining some emotional distance from their overwhelming memories. Our research (van der Kolk and Ducey 1989) has shown that traumatized people have a decreased capacity for analyzing and planning. This may be related to a relative inactivity in the left hemisphere, particularly the language area, and heightened activity in the right limbic system in PTSD (Rauch et al. 1996). One can conceptualize the work of stabilization as helping maximize frontal lobe activity by learning to observe and attend, thereby diminishing the power of trauma-related physical sensations, emotions, and perceptions.

Marsha Linehan (1993) called the prime psychological resource that allows people mastery over physiological arousal *mindfulness.* People need to learn to observe and to describe their feelings and reactions without applying judgment (idealization of devaluation) or without immediately seeking relief. The task of development is what Jean Piaget called *decentration:* learning to attend to one's emotions, even if they are distressing, and accepting feelings for what they are. Traumatized patients need to learn to uncouple trauma-related physical sensations from reactivating trauma-related emotion and perceptions. They need to learn to distinguish between their internal sensations and the external events that precipitated them. In addition, they need to learn how to articulate plans of action that can predictably help them to alter the way they feel.

As long as the trauma is experienced in the form of speechless terror, the body tends to continue to react to conditional stimuli as a return of the trauma, without the capacity to define alternative courses of action. However, when the triggers are identified and the individual gains the capacity to attach words to somatic experiences, these stimuli lose some of their terror (Harber and Pennebaker 1992). Thus, the task of therapy is both to create a capacity to be mindful of current experience and to create symbolic representations of past traumatic experiences with the goal of uncoupling physical sensations from trauma-based emotional responses, thereby taming the associated terror.

Any decrease in the intensity and duration of hyperarousal states (alarm or dissociation) will decrease the probability of experiencing trauma-related flashbacks and the resulting self-destructive acting out. For this stabilization to occur, safety and predictability are key elements. Patients need to develop an internal locus of control by understanding and managing uncomfortable sensations and emotions and by learning effective plans of action.

Intrusive recollections of the trauma come in many different forms. Many people fail to realize that "flashbacks" are not just visual and often lack a narrative component. Flashbacks are fragmented sensory experiences involving affective, visual, tactile, gustatory, olfactory, auditory, and motor systems (van der Kolk and Fisler 1995). Without a visual image to anchor an experience as belonging to past tactile, affective, kinesthetic, or olfactory sensory fragments, traumatized individuals are prone to experience the flashback as belonging to the present. Stabilization consists of learning how to correctly interpret the intrusive sensory fragments of traumatic experience.

As long as patients are prone to dissociatively reexperience such fragments of their traumas, passively listening and making meaning can be counterproductive. It is critical to label what is going on and help patients understand and process these somatic experiences. In this context it is useful to reframe many of the patients' behaviors as symptoms of feeling overwhelmed by the physical sensations associated with their trauma: self-destructive impulses, hypervigilance, self-loathing, and shame. They usually can be understood either as trauma-related physical or emotional states or as old, misguided attempts to cope with overwhelming situations. Under stress, these patients tend to regress to how they felt at a time when the people who were supposed to take care of them actually were the sources of fear and anxiety. They cannot teach themselves how to be safe, because many of them simply lack a baseline understanding of what that means.

Affective hyperarousal can effectively be treated with the judicious use of serotonin reuptake inhibitors and emotion-regulation training, which consists of identifying, labeling, and altering emotional states. Patients are encouraged to attend to the sensory details of their experiences, locating where they feel the sensations associated with emotional states in their bodies. This supports them to learn to identify the internal sources of their distress and tolerate them, as they observe that bodily sensations change over time. Gradually, patients learn to observe—rather than to run away from—the way they feel, and to plan alternative coping strategies. As long as chronically traumatized people have not learned these skills, they tend to feel desperately dependent on people in their environment, which makes it difficult for them to question and disagree with people they feel are essential for their survival.

All discussions between patients and therapists must include close attention to the effects of particular actions—such as work, relationships, and recreational activities—on their capacity to feel in control and free from triggers for PTSD symptoms. Patients need to practice stabilization techniques, which can help them ground themselves when they feel hyperaroused or dissociated. These techniques can include changing postures and noticing the sensation of feeling one's feet on the floor, or looking around the room and identifying familiar objects. It is useful to access several different sensory modalities—tactile, visual, or auditory stimuli—such as touching cold objects like stones or ice cubes or smelling coffee or tea.

Resource Identification and Installation

PTSD symptoms should not be treated until the available internal and external resources have been identified and are in place: skills and hobbies, activities that calm the patient down and that give satisfaction and a sense of competence. For most people, feelings of interpersonal safety are essential to provide the sense of inner calm to make a distinction between current situations and the roots of current distress in the past. Fear needs to be tamed for people to be able to think clearly and be conscious of what they currently need. For this it is necessary to have a body with predictable and controllable reactions to daily hassles. Developing a sense of bodily mastery and competence contradicts an identity of physical helplessness. In our program we actively encourage our patients to expose themselves to situations that precipitate a certain amount of controllable anxiety and that include a great deal of social support. Programs such as "model mugging" and Outward Bound can be immensely helpful to create physical and sensate memories of mastery. Having such experiences helps patients to associate certain anxiety-provoking physical sensations not only with traumatic memories but also with feelings of mastery, competence, and triumph.

Use of Language and the Creation of Narratives

Putting one's daily experiences, emotions, and observations into words is one important element of posttraumatic therapy. Language creates the capacity to generate complex internal representations of one's reality. This promotes gaining a certain emotional distance from the trauma and observing the experiences from a variety of analytical vantage points. Language is indispensable for communicating the totality of one's experiences and distress. Uncommunicated experience tends to lead to emotional isolation—a sense of being forsaken and no longer part of the human race. In contrast, feeling understood and amplifying what one knows and understands by communicating with others (in this case the therapist) is one of the great joys of being human.

Putting an experience into words is one way in which people can regain the capacity to imagine alternative outcomes, besides the disaster of the trauma. Of course, the study of how children process upsetting experiences has taught us that drawing and play acting are their preferred modes of coping with distressing experiences. Child therapists have learned those lessons well and have applied them in their consulting rooms. Some imaginative therapists who work with traumatized adults have successfully adapted those techniques for work with their adult patients.

Over time, as patients learn to recount what is happening in their lives and how they feel about it, they come to understand how they engage in repetitive patterns of distress, failure to communicate, and maladaptive behaviors—such as self-mutilation, use of alcohol and drugs, and impulsive aggressive and sexual behaviors—as ways of dealing with specific trauma-related sensations, affects, and impulses. Learning how to observe themselves, they come to "own" these reactions as occurring in response to certain actions and reactions to and by bosses, coworkers, lovers, children, and therapists, but changing the behaviors of the people who precipitate these reactions cannot set them free from their own exaggerated responses. Understanding these patterns of distress and making connections between internal states and self-destructive ways of coping with them is the essence of dynamic psychotherapy. Understanding how these patterns are often rooted in ways of coping with an unresolved past helps identify particular sensations that remain in need of further "processing."

Trauma Processing

The key aspects of the treatment of traumatic memories are described differently by different therapeutic schools. Most clinicians and researchers believe that for traumatic memories to lose their emotional valence, the patients must be confronted with new information that is incompatible with the rigid traumatic memory. According to Rothbaum and Foa (1996), two conditions are required for the reduction of fear, and hence for the treatment of PTSD: 1) the person must attend to trauma-related information in a manner that will activate his or her own traumatic memories, and 2) the context needs to directly contradict major elements of the trauma, such as feeling safe. The decrease of fear or anxiety depends on the controlled and coordinated evocation of environmental trauma-related cues, the sensory and motoric responses, and the meaning of the traumatic memory. Thus, the critical issue is to expose the patient to an experience that contains elements that are sufficiently similar to the trauma to activate it and that at the same time contains aspects that are incompatible enough to change it. This eventually is supposed to lead to desensitization. Other chapters in this volume demonstrate that this technique can be helpful for many traumatized individuals.

Exposing trauma victims too directly to their memories runs the risk of precipitating hyperarousal and sensitization, a common clinical occurrence that was well documented in the research on exposure treatment by Pitman et al. (1991). Thus, treatment should avoid the full-blown reactivation of the pain, dissociation, and helplessness associated with the trauma in general and of earlier interpersonal betrayal within the therapeutic relationship in particular. Effective treatment should minimize the time spent on reliving the past with its concomitant emotional devastation and should instead help patients to be fully present in the here now without the residual dissociation and/or hyperarousal characteristic of PTSD.

In our clinic we principally use eye movement desensitization and reprocessing (EMDR) to help patients "process" their traumatic memories. We also use EMDR for "resource installation," by amplifying memories and sensations of safe or pleasant experiences in the patient's mind. Despite its unconventional method, EMDR has been the subject of controlled studies involving well over 200 subjects, more than any single psychopharmacologic or psychological intervention for PTSD (Chemtob et al. 2000). EMDR is predicated on the notion that experiences are stored in memory networks that are organized by affect and that contain related memories, thoughts, images, emotions, and sensations. The storage of traumatic information is fragmentary and is usually intensely distressing. It is thought that EMDR facilitates rapid adaptive, associative information processing by integrating sensations, affects, and self-attributions. In this way, it may share some of the same qualities as REM sleep, which has been posited to help process distressing day-to-day experiences (Stickgold 1998). However, at this point there is no scientific evidence of why EMDR works.

The use of EMDR has several advantages over the more conventional exposure techniques. These include the fact that it is easier to "dose": the moment that a patient experiences emotional arousal he or she is asked to "stay there" and to process the memory while engaging in eye movements. This helps the patient avoid the extremes of physiologic arousal that so often accompanies full-blown exposure therapy. By tracking merely emotional shifts and asking the patient to name the somatic sensations that accompany those shifts, one permits the patient not to communicate precisely what is upsetting. Being able to avoid telling what is going on has major advantages. Trauma by definition involves "speechless terror": patients often are simply unable to put what they feel into words and are left with intense emotions simply without being able to articulate what is going on. For many traumatized individuals the experience is contaminated by shame and guilt, which may keep them from wanting to communicate what they are thinking. Respecting the patients' privacy while still being able to process the associated memories takes away the potential of an unnecessary voyeuristic element in the therapeutic relationship.

Flooding and exposure are by no means harmless treatment techniques: exposure to information consistent with a traumatic memory can be expected to strengthen anxiety (i.e., sensitize and thereby aggravate PTSD symptoms). Excessive arousal may make the PTSD patient worse by interfering with the acquisition of new information (Strian and Klicpera 1978). When that occurs, the traumatic memories will not be corrected but will merely be confirmed; instead of promoting habituation, the treatment may accidentally foster sensitization.

Conclusions

Given the prevalence of chronic complex trauma in psychiatric patients, it is astounding how little research has been done on this population. Much of the existing knowledge comes from a reframing of the diagnosis of borderline personality disorder (BPD) as a disorder related to childhood abuse and neglect (Herman et al. 1989; Zanarini et al. 1997). Most research on the treatment of that disorder, such as that conducted by Marsha Linehan, has largely ignored the traumatic origins of BPD and instead has focused on symptom stabilization. Research on BPD has carried much of the same stigma that has always accompanied research on hysteria, the historical precursor of both BPD and complex PTSD. In fact, much of the current understanding of the treatment of this disorder has its origin in the writings on hysteria by Janet (1889/1973, 1919/1925) and by Freud (1896/1962; Breuer and Freud 1893/1955). Both of these early clinicians placed the traumatic origins of this disorder central in their treatment approaches. Both ran onto considerable opposition and academic difficulties while studying the best treatments for these patients. Janet persisted and went into oblivion, Freud disavowed the study of trauma and became the defining figure of twentieth-century psychiatry. Clearly, although the study of neuroses caused by war, motor vehicle accidents, hurricanes, and other noninterpersonal traumas has become respectable, investigating that darkest side of human nature—our capacity to horribly abuse and neglect our own offspring and intimates—continues to be rife with controversy.

Because so little systematic research has been done on these patients, many questions remain about what constitutes optimal treatment. Some writers (Herman 1992; McCann and Pearlman 1992) emphasize the importance of a restorative therapeutic relationship, whereas others (e.g., van der Kolk 1996b) have been concerned about reenactment of traumatic relationships within the therapy and emphasize the building of coping skills, the formation of loose associations (in which a particular sensation loses its power to evoke entire traumatic scenes and the patient learns to attach new meanings to old sensations), and the processing of traumatic memories. Perhaps what is most important for these patients is to learn to have a subjective sense of mastery and competence that will allow them to live in the present without being constantly pulled back into experiencing the present as a recurrence of the past.

Clearly, now that the long-term psychological and biological consequences of early interpersonal trauma are beginning to be spelled out in as much detail as they have in the past few years, the need for adequate treatment outcome research has become critical. Up until the present, very little funding has been available for such research, leaving the field to rely on clinical wisdom and vehement doctrinal disagreements.

References

Ackerman PT, Newton JEO, McPherson WB, et al: Prevalence of post traumatic stress disorder and other psychiatric diagnoses in three groups of abused children (sexual, physical, and both). Child Abuse Negl 22(8):759–774, 1998

American Psychiatric Association: Diagnostic and Statistical Manual of Mental Disorders, 3rd Edition. Washington, DC, American Psychiatric Association, 1980

Archibald HC, Tuddenham RD: Persistent stress reaction after combat: a 20-year follow-up. Arch Gen Psychiatry 12(5):1–30, 1965

Beitchman JH, Zucker KJ, Hood JE, et al: A review of the long-term effects of child sexual abuse. Child Abuse Negl 16(1):101–118, 1992

Bremner JD, Southwick SM, Johnson DR, et al: Childhood physical abuse and combat-related posttraumatic stress disorder in Vietnam veterans. Am J Psychiatry 150(2):235–239, 1993

Breuer J, Freud S: Studies on hysteria (1893–1895), in The Standard Edition of the Complete Psychological Works of Sigmund Freud, Vol 3. Translated and edited by Strachey J. London, Hogarth Press, 1955, pp 1–305

Briere JN: Therapy for Adults Molested as Children: Beyond Survival, 2nd Edition. New York, Springer, 1996

Brown D, Fromm E: Hypnotherapy and Hypnoanalysis. Hillsdale, NJ, Lawrence Erlbaum, 1986

Brown D, Scheflin AW, Hammond DC: Memory, Trauma Treatment, and the Law. New York, WW Norton, 1998

Burgess AW, Holmstrom LL: Rape trauma syndrome. Am J Psychiatry 131(9):981–986, 1974

Chemtob CM, Tolin DF, van der Kolk BA, et al: Eye movement desensitization and reprocessing, in Effective Treatments for PTSD: Practice Guidelines From the International Society for Traumatic Stress Studies. Edited by Foa EB, Keane TM, Friedman MJ. New York, Guilford, 2000, pp 333–335

Chilcoat HD, Breslau N: Posttraumatic stress disorder and drug disorders: testing causal pathways. Arch Gen Psychiatry 55(10):913–917, 1998

Chu JA: Rebuilding Shattered Lives: The Responsible Treatment of Complex Post-Traumatic and Dissociative Disorders. New York, Wiley, 1998

Cicchetti D, Carlson V: Child Maltreatment: Theory and Research on the Causes and Consequences of Child Abuse and Neglect. New York, Cambridge University Press, 1989

Cicchetti D, Toth SL: Developmental psychopathology and disorders of affect, in Developmental Psychopathology, Vol 2: Risk, Disorder, and Adaptation. Wiley Series on Personality Processes. Edited by Cicchetti D, Cohen DJ. New York, Wiley, 1995, pp 369–420

Cole PM, Putnam FW: Effect of incest on self and social functioning: developmental psychopathology perspective. J Consult Clin Psychol 60(2):174–184, 1992

Courtois CA: Theory, sequencing, and strategy in treating adult survivors. New Dir Mental Health Serv 51:47–60, 1991

Crittenden PM: Distorted patterns of relationship in maltreating families: the role of internal representational models. Journal of Reproductive and Infant Psychology 6:183–189, 1988

DeGroot JM, Kennedy S, Rodin G, et al: Correlates of sexual abuse in women with anorexia nervosa and bulimia nervosa. Can J Psychiatry 37(7):516–518, 1992

Drossman DA, Leserman J, Nachman G, et al: Sexual and physical abuse in women with functional or organic gastrointestinal disorders. Ann Intern Med 113(11):828–833, 1990

Ehlers A, Clark DM, Dunmore E, et al: Predicting response to exposure treatment in PTSD: the role of mental defeat and alienation. J Trauma Stress 11(3):457–471, 1998

Felitti VJ, Anda RF, Nordernberg D, et al: Relationship of childhood abuse to many of the leading causes of death in adults: the Adverse Childhood Experiences (ACE) Study. Am J Prev Med 14(4):245–258, 1998

Field T: Attachment as psychobiological attunement: being on the same wavelength, in The Psychobiology of Attachment and Separation. Edited by Reite M, Fields T. Orlando, FL, Academic, 1985

Foa EB, Riggs DS, Massie ED, et al: The impact of fear activation and anger on the efficacy of exposure treatment for posttraumatic stress disorder. Behav Ther 26(3):487–499, 1995

Foa EB, Cashman L, Jaycox LH, et al: The validation of a self-report measure of posttraumatic stress disorder: the Posttraumatic Diagnostic Scale. Psychol Assess 9(4):445–451, 1997

Ford JD: Disorders of extreme stress following war-zone military trauma: associated features of posttraumatic stress disorder or comorbid but distinct syndromes. J Consult Clin Psychol 67(1):3–12, 1999

Ford JD, Kidd TP: Early childhood trauma and disorders of extreme stress as predictors of treatment outcome with chronic posttraumatic stress disorder. J Trauma Stress 11(4):743–761, 1998

Ford JD, Fisher P, Larson L: Object relations as a predictor of treatment outcome with chronic posttraumatic stress disorder. J Consult Clin Psychol 65(4):547–559, 1997

Freedman AM, Kaplan HI, Sadock BJ: Modern Synopsis of Comprehensive Textbook of Psychiatry. Baltimore, MD, Williams & Wilkins, 1972

Freud S: Formulations on the two principles of mental functioning (1911), in The Standard Edition of the Complete Psychological Works of Sigmund Freud, Vol 12. Translated and edited by Strachey J. London, Hogarth Press, 1959

Freud S: The Aetiology of Hysteria (1896), in The Standard Edition of the Complete Psychological Works of Sigmund Freud, Vol. 3. Translated and edited by Strachey J. London, Hogarth Press, 1962, pp 189–222

Gendlin ET: Focusing-Oriented Psychotherapy: A Manual of the Experiential Method. New York, Guilford, 1998

Golding JM, Stein JA, Siegel JM, et al: Sexual assault history and use of health and mental health services. Am J Community Psychol 16(5):625–644, 1988

Harber KD, Pennebaker JW: Overcoming traumatic memories, in The Handbook of Emotion and Memory: Research and Theory. Edited by Christianson SA. Hillsdale, NJ, Erlbaum, 1992, pp 359–386

Herman JL: Trauma and Recovery. New York, Basic Books, 1992

Herman JL, Perry JC, van der Kolk BA: Childhood trauma in borderline personality disorder. Am J Psychiatry 146(4):490–495, 1989

Herzog DB, Staley JE, Carmody S, et al: Childhood sexual abuse in anorexia nervosa and bulimia nervosa: a pilot study. J Am Acad Child Adolesc Psychiatry 32(5):962–966, 1993

Horowitz MJ: Stress response syndromes: character style and dynamic psychotherapy Arch Gen Psychiatry 6:768–781, 1974

Horowitz MJ, Solomon GF: Delayed stress response syndromes in Vietnam veterans, in Stress Disorders Among Vietnam Veterans: Theory, Research and Treatment. Edited by Figley CR. New York, Brunner/Mazel, 1978, pp 268–280

Janet P: L'automatisme psychologique: essai de psychologie experimentale sur les formes inferieures de l'activite humaine (1889). Paris, Felix Alcan, 1973

Janet P: Psychological Healing (1919), Vol. 1–2. Translated by Paul C, Paul E. New York, Macmillan, 1925

Kardiner A: The Traumatic Neuroses of War. New York, Paul B Hoeber, 1941

Kendall-Tackett KA, Williams LM, Finkelhor D: Impact of sexual abuse on children: a review and synthesis of recent empirical studies. Psychol Bull 113(1): 164–180, 1993

Kernberg OF: Borderline Syndromes and Pathological Narcissism. Northvale, NJ, Jason Aronson, 1975

Kluft RP: Clinical presentations of multiple personality disorder. Psychiatr Clin North Am 14(3):605–629, 1991

Kluft RP: The use of hypnosis with dissociative disorders. Psychiatric Medicine 10(4):31–46, 1992

Krystal H: Trauma and affects. Psychoanal Study Child 33:81–116, 1978

Levine PA, Frederick A: Waking the Tiger—Healing Trauma: The Innate Capacity to Transform Overwhelming Experiences. Berkeley, CA, USA North Atlantic Books, 1997

Linehan MM: Cognitive-Behavioral Treatment of Borderline Personality Disorder. New York, Guilford, 1993

Macy R: Unpublished doctoral dissertation, Mount Union College, Alliance, OH, 2002

McCann IL, Pearlman LA: Constructivist self-development theory: a theoretical framework for assessing and treating traumatized college students. J Am Coll Health 40(4):189–196, 1992

McDonagh-Coyle A, McHugo G, Ford J, et al: Cognitive-behavioral treatment for childhood sexual abuse survivors with PTSD. Paper presented at the 15th Annual Meeting of the International Society for Traumatic Stress Studies, Miami, Florida, November 1999

McFarlane AC, McFarlane CM, Gilchrist PN: Posttraumatic bulimia and anorexia nervosa. Int J Eat Disord 7(5):705–708, 1988

Moeller TP, Bachmann GA, Moeller JR: The combined effects of physical, sexual, and emotional abuse during childhood: long-term health consequences for women. Child Abuse Negl 17:623–640, 1993

Ogata SN, Silk KR, Goodrich S, et al: Childhood sexual and physical abuse in adult patients with borderline personality disorder. Am J Psychiatry 147(8):1008–1013, 1990

Pelcovitz D, van der Kolk BA, Roth SH, et al: Development of a criteria set and a structured interview for disorders of extreme stress (SIDES). J Trauma Stress 10(1):3–16, 1997

Pesso A, Crandell J (eds): Moving Psychotherapy: Theory and Application of Pesso System/Psychomotor Therapy. Cambridge, MA, Brookline Books, 1991

Pitman RK, Altman B, Greenwald E, et al: Psychiatric complications during flooding therapy for posttraumatic stress disorder. J Clin Psychiatry 52:17–20, 1991

Polusny MA, Follette VM: Long-term correlates of child sexual abuse: theory and review of the empirical literature. Applied and Preventive Psychology 4(3): 143–166, 1995

Porges S: The polyvagal theory of emotions. Psychoneuroendocrinology 23:837–845, 1998

Putnam FW: Pierre Janet and modern views of dissociation. J Trauma Stress 2(4): 413–429, 1989

Putnam FW: Dissociation in Children and Adolescents: A Developmental Perspective. New York, Guilford, 1997

Putnam FW: Childhood maltreatment adverse outcomes. Paper presented at the 152nd Annual Meeting of the American Psychiatric Association, Washington, DC, May 15–20, 1999

Pynoos RS, Steinberg AM, Goenjian A: Traumatic stress in childhood and adolescence: recent developments and current controversies, in Traumatic Stress: The Effects of Overwhelming Experience on Mind, Body, and Society. Edited by van der Kolk BA, McFarlane AC, Weisaeth L. New York, Guilford, 1996

Rapkin BD, Mulvey EP, Maton KI, et al: Criteria of excellence, III: methods of studying community psychology, in Researching Community Psychology: Issues of Theory and Methods. Edited by Tolan P, Keys C. Washington, DC, American Psychological Association, 1990, pp 147–167

Rauch SL, van der Kolk BA, Fisler RE, et al: A symptom provocation study of posttraumatic stress disorder using positron emission tomography and script-driven imagery. Arch Gen Psychiatry 53(5):380–387, 1996

Reich R: Character Analysis [Character Analyse]. New York, Basic Books, 1937

Rodriguez N, Ryan SW, Vande Kemp H, et al: Posttraumatic stress disorder in adult female survivors of childhood sexual abuse: a comparison study. J Consult Clin Psychol 65(1):53–59, 1997

Ross CA, Norton GR, Wozney K: Multiple personality disorder: an analysis of 236 cases. Can J Psychiatry 34(5):413–418, 1989

Ross CA, Miller SD, Bjornson L, et al: Abuse histories in 102 cases of multiple personality disorder. Can J Psychiatry 36(2):97–101, 1991

Roth SH, Newman E, Pelcovitz D, et al: Complex PTSD in victims exposed to sexual and physical abuse: results from the DSM-IV Field Trial for Posttraumatic Stress Disorder. J Trauma Stress 10(4):539–555, 1997

Rothbaum BO, Foa EB: Cognitive-behavioral therapy for posttraumatic stress disorder, in Traumatic Stress: The Effects of Overwhelming Experience on Mind, Body, and Society. Edited by van der Kolk BA, McFarlane AC, Weisaeth L. New York, Guilford, 1996, pp 491–509

Saxe GN, van der Kolk BA, Berkowitz R, et al: Dissociative disorders in psychiatric inpatients. Am J Psychiatry 150(7):1037–1042, 1993

Saxe GN, Chinman G, Berkowitz R, et al: Somatization in patients with dissociative disorders. Am J Psychiatry 151(9):1329–1334, 1994

Schachtel EG: On memory and childhood amnesia. Psychiatry 10:1–26, 1947

Stern D: The Interpersonal World of the Infant. New York, Basic Books, 1985

Stickgold R: REM, memory, PTSD, and EMDR. Article presented at the EMDR International Association, Annual Conference, Baltimore, MD, 1998

Strian F, Klicpera C: Significance of autonomic arousal for the development and persistence of anxiety states. Nervenarzt 49(10):576–583, 1978

van der Kolk BA (ed): Psychological Trauma. Washington, DC, American Psychiatric Press, 1987, pp 1–30 van der Kolk BA, Ducey C: The psychological processing of traumatic experience: Rorschach patterns in PTSD. J Trauma Stress 2:259–274, 1989

van der Kolk BA, Fisler RE: Dissociation and the fragmentary nature of traumatic memories: overview and exploratory study. J Trauma Stress 8(4):505–525, 1995

van der Kolk BA, Perry C, Herman JL: Childhood origins of self-destructive behavior. Am J Psychiatry 148:1665–1671, 1991

van der Kolk BA, Dreyfuss D, Berkowitz R, et al: Fluoxetine in posttraumatic stress. J Clin Psychiatry 55:517–522, 1994

van der Kolk BA, McFarlane AC, van der Hart O: A general approach to treatment of posttraumatic stress disorder, in Traumatic Stress: The Effects of Overwhelming Experience on Mind, Body, and Society. Edited by van der Kolk BA, McFarlane AC, Weisaeth L. New York, Guilford, 1996a, pp 417–440

van der Kolk BA, McFarlane AC, Weisaeth L (eds): Traumatic Stress: The Effects of Overwhelming Experience on Mind, Body, and Society. New York, Guilford, 1996b, pp 559–575

van der Kolk BA, van der Hart O, Marmar CR: Dissociation and information processing in posttraumatic stress disorder, in Traumatic Stress: The Effects of Overwhelming Experience on Mind, Body and Society. Edited by van der Kolk BA, McFarlane AC, Weisaeth L. New York, Guilford, 1996c, pp 303–327

Walker LE: Battered women and learned helplessness. Victimology 2(suppl 4):525–534, 1977/1978

Wang CT, Daro D: Current Trends in Child Abuse Reporting and Fatalities: The Results of the 1997 Annual Fifty State Survey. Center on Child Abuse Prevention Research, National Committee to Prevent Child Abuse, Washington, DC, 1997

Westen D, Lohr N, Silk KR, et al: Object relations and social cognition in borderlines, major depressives, and normals: a thematic apperception test analysis. Psychol Assess 2(4):355–364, 1990a

Westen D, Ludolph P, Block MJ, et al: Developmental history and object relations in psychiatrically disturbed adolescent girls. Am J Psychiatry 147(8):1061–1068, 1990b

Widom CS: Childhood victimization and the development of personality disorders: unanswered questions remain. Arch Gen Psychiatry 56(7):607–608, 1999

Zanarini MC, Williams AA, Lewis RE, et al: Reported pathological childhood experiences associated with the development of borderline personality disorder. Am J Psychiatry 154(8):1101–1106, 1997

7

Treating Survivors in the Immediate Aftermath of Traumatic Events

Arieh Y. Shalev, M.D.

Several factors make it extremely difficult to describe and discuss the treatment of survivors in the immediate aftermath of traumatic events. At such times, the survivor's actual needs may be very urgent; secondary stressors may still be operating; expressions of distress are volatile and highly reactive to external realities; and symptoms expressed may not reflect psychopathology. Importantly, normal healing processes are already operating, and significant assistance is being provided by natural supporters and healers (e.g., relatives, community leaders) and should not be interfered with. Professional helpers are often enduring significant stress themselves and do not operate in their usual environment. The adequacy of both the medical and psychological treatment models must therefore be questioned. An alternative model may be considered—one that favors knowledge of pathogenic processes over symptom recognition. The treatment of early survivors requires therapeutic flexibility. The more one is professionally prepared to handle novelty and uncertainty, the better one's therapeutic impact. Furthermore, helpers' unavoidable distress should be managed during the intervention, such that they remain effective and avoid causing harm to themselves.

Current knowledge of posttraumatic stress disorder (PTSD) has sensi-

tized the public and the mental health community to the damaging potential
of exposure to traumatic events. From a clinical point of view, it is important
to note that most trauma survivors who develop prolonged stress disorders
show symptoms of distress in the early aftermath of traumatization (Rothbaum
and Foa 1993). Moreover, most instances of recovery from early and distressful
responses to traumatic events occur within the following year (Kessler et al.
1995; Shalev et al. 1997). The early aftermath of traumatization therefore
offers a window of opportunity during which individuals at risk for developing
chronic stress disorders can be identified and treated (Bryant et al. 1998; Foa
et al.1995; Z. Solomon and Benbenishty 1986).

The optimal time for such interventions, however, is unclear. On one
hand, the very early days that follow traumatic events may constitute a
"critical" or "sensitive" period, during which neuronal plasticity is
enhanced (Shalev 1999) and indelible aversive learning occurs (Shalev et
al.1992). On the other hand, most trauma survivors do not present to treatment before having endured weeks of suffering, possibly because they (and
others around them) see the initial distress and the associated symptoms as
a normal response. It is also unclear whether the very early and short interventions, such as onsite debriefing, have any prolonged effect (Bisson and
Deahl 1994; Deahl et al. 2000; Mayou et al. 2000; Raphael et al. 1996; Rose
et al. 1999). Studies of early treatment of combat soldiers, however, point
to a more positive outcome (S.D. Solomon et al. 1992; Z. Solomon and
Benbenishty 1986).

Beyond the optimal timing, the content and techniques of immediate
interventions must be examined. Interventions conducted weeks or months
after trauma have received some attention in the literature and involve
treatment techniques that resemble those used in prolonged mental disorders (e.g., cognitive-behavioral therapy). Whether or not the earlier, acute
interventions should be conducted according to the same principles is
unclear. What is clear, however, is that at the end of the impact phase of a
trauma the physical and mental condition of survivors is very different from
that seen days or a few weeks later. Most are midway between enduring
stress and reappraising its consequences (Lazarus and Folkman 1984).
Helpers and therapists who approach the survivors at this stage are also "in
the field" and not in their usual working environment. Some are experiencing, along with their clients, a major life event. As such, these circumstances suggest a modified approach.

There are several ways in which therapy during the acute phase may be
different. First, a conceptual reframing is needed: at this phase one may still
be handling the trauma, rather than treating a posttraumatic condition.
Psychological rescue (or first aid) may therefore be a proper term for some
interventions. Second, along with symptoms, current sources of stress

should be in the forefront of the clinical evaluation. Relocation, separation, or continuous threat (such as during political repression) are powerful modulators of behavior that cannot be ignored when the totality of the individual is considered. Help at this stage may consist of mitigating the effect of concurrent stressors. Third, the complexity of events and responses should be noted: The mental and physical conditions that follow traumatic events are extremely complex, and the resulting behavior is unstable and rapidly changing (Rosser and Dewar 1991; Shalev et al. 1993; Yitzhaki et al. 1991). The perception of the event may vary from one individual to another (Shalev et al. 1993). For better or worse, individuals may be suggestible and unusually reactive; they may be very responsive to the emotional tone of helpers but also reactive to real or fantasized realities, such as rumors. Fourth, expressions of distress are often appropriate at this stage, and one should be very careful not to classify them as symptoms in the sense of being indicative of a mental disorder. Medicalizing (or pathologizing) an early response is often the result of profound misunderstanding of the role of pain and anxiety as signals to the body, the psyche, and others. An essential diagnostic element, at this stage, is therefore not so much the intensity, but rather the appropriateness and the "productiveness" of the early response in engaging a healing process. Fifth, during rescue efforts, professionals and nonprofessionals may have similar roles (e.g., soothing, comforting, orienting, reassuring). Nonprofessionals, however, are available in larger numbers and include the survivor's natural supporters (e.g., relatives, peers) and other community members. These supporters may also be overwhelmed and distressed, and in many instances the role of the professional helper is to support and guide the supporters (e.g., nurses, family members, disaster area managers). Finally, sharing another human being's grief is a powerful emotional response, which has a unique healing power. Sharing may also be painful. Sharing by therapists, therefore, is both desirable and unavoidable. The degree to which professional helpers are induced to share emotions, are able to sustain such experiences, and receive adequate preparation and support in so doing may have important effects on their efficacy as helpers and on their own well-being.

The above-mentioned particulars of the early response to traumatic events lead to asking another important question: Who, if at all, should be treated by mental health specialists? On the one hand, the very frequent occurrence of traumatic events (Breslau and Davis 1992) defies any effort to provide specialized care for all. This is especially true for underdeveloped countries and major disaster areas. Moreover, as mentioned above, in most cases the responses are self-limited. Yet, given the risk that survivors will develop chronic stress disorders, providing such help may make the difference between recovery and life-long illness.

This dilemma has been approached in two systematic ways. The first was to provide specialized treatment to those identified as being ill (e.g., soldiers who ceased to function during combat because of stress responses) (Kormos 1978; Z. Solomon 1993). The second consisted of covering all those exposed by providing some professional intervention, recently in the form of debriefing. Far from being solved, however, the question of whether or not to intervene, or what kind of intervention to provide, emerges again and again in each individual case. Deciding what to do and how much is the essence of clinical wisdom. This chapter proposes to assist in such decisions by pointing to the following ideas:

- The dichotomous choice between treatment and no treatment should be replaced by the notion of *depth of treatment.*
- The early and urgent needs of all should be addressed (although not necessarily by psychological interventions).
- Trauma survivors should be considered as being at risk for developing traumatic stress disorders.
- Specific risk factors should be evaluated, for each case, on the basis of the existing literature.
- The survivors' progress toward recovery should be followed and clinical decisions made on the basis of longitudinal observations (instead of cross-sectional examination).
- Treatment should be provided in the context of continuity of care.

This chapter delineates the implementation of these ideas. It starts by discussing the nature of traumatic events and subsequently outlines a framework for assessing trauma survivors. It then points to the general rules of early intervention and to some intervention techniques. It ends by advising clinicians regarding termination of treatment or continuity of care. To remain practical, the chapter avoids extended discussion of each point, instead directing the reader to the relevant literature.

Defining Trauma

DSM-IV (American Psychiatric Association 1994, p. 431) defines a traumatic event as including an element of threat ("actual or threatened death or serious injury, or a threat to the physical integrity of self or others") and a typical response ("intense fear, helplessness, or horror"). The DSM-IV definition sets an entry criterion for considering an event as traumatic in the context of making a diagnosis of PTSD. It should not be read, however, as a good enough descriptor of traumatic events; it is nonspecific (i.e., it applies to a wide variety of events from automobile accidents to incarceration in a concentration camp). Importantly, the DSM-IV definition does not address the mechanisms of mental traumatization.

Understanding the mechanisms of mental traumatization is extremely important, particularly when one's role is to evaluate and assist the recent survivor. Phenomenology alone is not enough at this stage; specific syndromes are not yet formed, there is great variability in the expression of distress, and one is better served by knowing the principles than by identifying sets of symptoms. Moreover, events are never "traumatic" just because they meet a threshold criterion. Extreme events become traumatic when they include one or several pathogenic elements or when the individual exposed is, for some reason, vulnerable to their effect.

This section outlines some of the traumatizing elements of events, the salient responses, and the ways in which people cope with traumatic stressors (and with their own responses). A discussion of vulnerability and risk factors for developing traumatic stress disorders is beyond the scope of this chapter.

Trauma Is More Than Fear and Threat

Although they were formerly believed to consist mainly of threat and fear response, extreme events may in fact traumatize people in many different ways. For some, fear and threat are indeed the essence of a trauma. For others, the traumatic event includes a major element of loss. Exposure to grotesque and disfigured human bodies may be the sole traumatizing element of some other events (McCarroll et al. 1995). Dehumanization, degradation, and humiliation are at the core of other experiences, such as rape, racially motivated trauma, and torture. Forced separation and relocation are other independent elements. For example, in a study of acute stress disorder among prisoners of a concentration camp (Kozaric et al. 1998), the prisoners rated lack of information about their families as the most stressful element of their captivity.

Several concrete elements of traumatic events are known to increase the risk of developing posttraumatic stress disorders. These include a threat to one's life and body integrity; severe physical harm or injury; receipt of intentional injury or harm; exposure to the grotesque; witnessing or learning of violence to loved ones; and causing the death of or severe harm to another (Green 1995).

The current inclusion of all such experiences under the title of psychological trauma implies that all of them are similar at some level (e.g., biologically). This, however, has not been proved convincingly. Indeed, specific ways in which one is traumatized may have a prolonged effect. A study of chronic PTSD, for example, suggests that exposure therapy, a method derived from a "threat and learning" model, may not be effective for survivors who have endured mental defeat, alienation, or permanent change (Ehlers et al. 1998a).

It follows that the clinical assessment of the recent survivor should clarify, first, what had been particularly traumatizing for an individual within the traumatic event. This is important because helpers may tend to assume a traumatizing element of an event by putting themselves (or their theory) in the place of the survivor. For example, assuming a priori that threat was the major traumatic element in the case of a survivor of a bombing or shooting incident: further inquiry may reveal other major sources of distress, such as having been separated from one's child during the evacuation or having failed to rescue significant others. Thus, in approaching the recent trauma survivor who is emerged in his or her particular narrative, understanding individual experience (as opposed to imposing one's own template) is the key for creating a therapeutic report.

Traumatic events can also be described by their psychological dimensions. Both psychologically and biologically, the severity of traumatic events is related to their being intense, inescapable, uncontrollable, and unexpected (Foa et al. 1992). Traumatic events can also be defined as those exceeding the person's coping resources (Lazarus and Folkman 1984) or breaking his or her protective defenses (Freud 1920/1957). In the assessment section below, it is made clear how these very abstract constructs may be used to guide one's practice.

The Biological Dimension

Construed under the general umbrella of stress and learned conditioning theories, the biological interpretation of mental traumatization has to explain the link between the early biological response to extreme events and the subsequent development of mental disorders. PTSD was originally explained as an exaggeration of a normal learning response, related to fear conditioning (Pitman 1988). The intensity of the initial adrenergic response was believed to foster emotional (and amygdala-mediated) learning, at the expense of rational or declarative, hippocampus-mediated learning (Metcalfe and Jacobs 1996). Accordingly, initial hypersecretion of the stress hormone epinephrine could be involved in an exaggeration and a consolidation of fear-related memories of the traumatic event (Cahill et al. 1994; McGaugh 1990). Supporting evidence for this theory can be found in a recent study, in which heart rate levels on admission to an emergency room after trauma were linked with the subsequent occurrence of PTSD (Shalev et al. 1998b).

Recently, the belief in a normal initial response has been challenged lcFarlane 1995; Yehuda et al. 1988). Abnormally low cortisol levels were reported shortly after trauma in individuals who were at higher risk for developing PTSD (Resnick et al. 1995; Yehuda et al.1990). A combination of increased adrenergic activation and low plasma levels of cortisol (Yehuda et al. 1990) had been shown to synergetically increase emotional learning (e.g., Munch et al. 1984).

An alternative model to the role of early biological responses argues that prolonged stress disorders result from factors that follow the initial exposure. PTSD, accordingly, follows a "progressive temporal sensitization" (Antelman 1988), which may be linked to the presence of persistent reminders of the traumatic event or to other stressors. Abnormal responses to startle, for example, do not develop in individuals with PTSD until 1–4 months after exposure (Shalev et al., in press). Recent prospective studies further suggest that depressive symptoms during the weeks that follow trauma are potent predictors of PTSD, which explains the occurrence of the disorder above and beyond predictions made from early symptoms of PTSD and anxiety (Freedman et al. 1999).

Possibly, a mixture of early stress responses and delayed activation of other biological cofactors is the best explanatory model for PTSD. Importantly, both theories point to the causal role of early distress in PTSD, hence the focus on reducing distress by all possible means.

Human Responses to Traumatic Stressors

Learning by Fear

Understanding the impact of threat and alarm on the brain comes from two theoretical bodies: stress theory and classical conditioning theory. Stress theory predicts that a threat would be responded to by specific innate or previously acquired defenses. Learned conditioning theory further predicts that stress would be associated with learning, particularly with learning avoidance and emotional memories.

The intensity of the threat (Resnick et al. 1995), its perception by the individual, and the quality of the immediate biopsychological response are therefore important predictors of subsequent psychopathology. The degree of control over events and over one's reaction is another important biopsychological modulator of the effect of stress on the brain (Prince and Anisman 1990). Physiologic stress (e.g., bleeding or dehydration) may further augment the hormonal stress response.

Impacted Grief

Beyond threat and fear, traumatic events often cause real and symbolic damage in the form of injury, separation or death of significant others, destruction of social networks, etc. Common to all of these is an element of loss. Loss is an independent and rather neglected dimension of mental traumatization (Hobfoll and Jackson 1991). Yet, far from being a secondary mechanism, loss and subsequent mental processing may be central to the development of PTSD. For example, loss of social network, due to relocation, was found to predict higher levels of PTSD symptoms 3–4 years after an earthquake (Bland et al. 1997). In fact, the core PTSD symptoms of intrusive recollections, numbing, and detachment were derived from earlier descriptions of unexpected loss (Lindemann 1994). The combined effect of loss and threat may similarly explain the frequent co-occurrence of PTSD and depression. Finally, responses to loss (e.g., of territory, offspring, or partners) may trigger independent neurobiological mechanisms of weaning and yearning, which may come to complement those related to threat.

Collapse of Structures and Defenses

A third traumatizing element of extreme events is the collapse of defensive mental structures. A frequent clinical expression of a breakdown of one's defenses is "I could not believe that this was happening" or "I felt paralyzed, unable to think and act." Breaking down, either during the event (e.g., surrender to pain or to a threat) or during the immediate aftermath may be extremely damaging to individuals in that previous defenses (or "coping mechanisms" or "cognitive schemata") are shattered (Janoff-Bulman 1989) and have to be rebuilt. This category of responses may be seen in exposure to human cruelty, forced degradation, trauma motivated by racism, human rights violations, and other events for which one cannot be mentally prepared. Again, being overwhelmed by grotesque events may be independent from experiencing a threat or a loss and yet may leave individuals puzzled, restless, and traumatized.

Isolation, Breakdown of Social Bonds

A most striking description of mental traumatization is that of an army officer who fought in the 1982 Lebanon war and developed PTSD. A few days into the war, while advancing on one of the main roads, the soldier and his men met an evacuation convoy, carrying casualties. Curious, the soldier stopped and jumped into one of the vehicles to discover the disfigured body of a mortally wounded close friend. He describes his experience in the following hours as follows: "From that point on nothing mattered any more. I continued to sit by my driver, as I did before, but was totally cut from others. I was completely alone, detached from my own soldiers who suddenly became total strangers to me." Dasberg (1976) described loneliness and social isolation as a core traumatic experience in combat stress reaction casualties of the 1956 Sinai campaign. Indeed, a piercing experience of many PTSD patients is the alienation from others, often expressed as "no one can ever understand what I have been through" (or what I am experiencing now).

Complementing these retrospective descriptions is the view that it is most difficult, if not impossible, to recover from trauma on one's own. As with serious physical injury, psychological wounds require the help of others to heal. The prime element of such help is to first break the wall of mental isolation that often follows exposure to extreme stressors—hence the importance of the quality of the initial contact established with survivors. It is equally important not to let such walls be built again: many trauma survivors carry the experience of good initial intent and subsequent "betrayal"—hence the importance of continuity of care.

Closing the Narrative

Finally, it is during the short period that follows trauma that a stable narrative of the traumatic events and of one's own responses is formed and consolidated (Shalev et al. 1998a), and these may shape the way in which the event will be remembered. Long-term memories of one's personal experience can often be confounded by what others have said and observed and by the larger social appraisal of the event (e.g., a failure, disaster, heroic act). Appraisal of one's current symptoms may predict PTSD above and beyond the effect of symptom severity (Ehlers et al. 1998b). The resulting mixture of personal and narrated facts is then consolidated into the "authentic" and "accurate" memory of the event. One is especially vulnerable to the effect of such interference during the immediate postevent period (Loftus 1993).

The Social Context

The social context of a traumatic event has major effects on the expression and the course of the immediate responses. Concrete and adverse social factors include the above-mentioned relocation, family disruption, and dissolution of communities. Other factors include community leadership and appraisal of the event by society. Societies tend to assign a value tag to being exposed to traumatic events and to one's behavior during exposure (e.g., merit, virtue, and honor versus shame, cowardice, or dishonor). These tags may confer a decisive meaning to the event, to which the survivor himself or herself may adhere. Importantly, the social perception of trauma survivors is often polarized, going from glorification to defamation. All too often it is the victim who is blamed for the victimizing event (e.g., a young woman who is blamed for having provoked a rape). Extreme social tags are often counterproductive. Both a recognized hero and a defamed coward may find it difficult to gain access to and work through their traumatic experiences. Those who intervene in the immediate aftermath of extreme events should therefore facilitate the expression of individual experiences and go beyond socially assigned value tags. One should let a hero cry out his or her fear and let a rape victim tell how wisely he or she managed to escape death.

Coping With Traumatic Stress

During the days that follow the traumatic event, trauma survivors go from a period of being under stress to a period of reappraisal and reevaluation. Typical for the "traumatic" period is the use of extreme defenses, such as overcontrol of emotions or dissociation and a focus on surviving trauma. The second period is characterized by intrusive recollections of the traumatic event and has for its main psychological task the assimilation of events and their consequences. Both periods can be extremely painful, hence the need to cope effectively during each of them. Following is a short description of the way in which coping can be assessed.

Coping can be defined as an effort to reduce the effect of environmental demands on physiologic and psychological responses, that is, "effort to increase the gap between stress and distress" (Pearlin 1978). Coping mechanisms have been authoritatively discussed (e.g., Lazarus and Folkman 1984), and most such descriptions address the myriad of specific ways in which people react to adversity. Individuals may indeed differ significantly in their preferred ways of coping: some are action prone, others are more reflective and analytical. Some express emotions, whereas others may hide them.

Studies of coping in trauma survivors have addressed the relative efficacy of specific ways of coping in cohorts of survivors (Z. Solomon et al. 1988). From a clinical point of view, however, what is ultimately important is the degree to which coping efforts are successful. In other words, in the immediate aftermath of traumatization the specific way in which the person copes with a stressor is often less important than the extent to which coping has been successful.

According to Pearlin and Schooler (1978), successful coping must protect four vital functions: 1) the ability to continue task-oriented activity, 2) the ability to regulate emotion, 3) the ability to sustain positive self-value, and 4) the capacity to maintain and enjoy rewarding interpersonal contacts. Importantly, effective coping may be seen despite extreme misery; and conversely, poor coping may follow events that objectively appear to be quite mild.

Symptoms Expressed After Trauma

Symptoms of Distress as an Effective Human Behavior

In their march toward recovery, trauma survivors express common responses that may enhance communication with others (e.g., by telling their story time and again), recruit support (e.g., by expressing a "cry for help"), and effectively initiate a process of learning and reappraisal (by going back to memories of the traumatic event and associating them with one's past experiences). In some cases, however, the same expressions may prevent communication (e.g., when telling the story if fearfully avoided or truncated), decrease the helping response of others, and consolidate the link between traumatic memories and negative emotions. In other words, the effectiveness of *expressed* behavior is most important (see Coping Efficacy, below). This section outlines the three common patterns of the early responses to trauma.

Symptoms Are Complex and Unstable

People react to traumatic events in many different ways. The intensity of the fear response may vary from fight or flight to freezing and surrender. Bodily responses, such as increased heart rate, are seen and may predict subsequent PTSD (Shalev et al. 1998b). Extreme psychological responses—such as dissociation, disorientation, and confusion—may also be seen and require specific management (Marmar et al. 1994). Some trauma survivors look sad, exhausted, and depressed. Physical injury and distress of physiologic origins (e.g., dehydration, hypothermia) are also seen and may be predictive of PTSD (Blanchard et al. 1997).

A study of combat stress reaction (CSR) in Israel found that symptoms expressed shortly after combat were "polymorphous and labile" (Yitzhaki et al. 1991). They included a mixture of exhaustion, stupefaction, sadness, anxiety, agitation, and blunted affect. These symptoms varied rapidly with time and in response to external reality. Another longitudinal observation found that initial heroic response in some survivors was often fostered by exposure to the media or by the need to be there for others (Shalev et al. 1993). To me, such behavior suggests that the survivor is still "within the trauma" and is using extreme defenses to cope with the event. These initial responses, however, do not last and are quickly replaced by the unavoidable circle of intrusive and painful recollections of the traumatic event.

Symptoms Are Normally Expressed, Yet Some Are Alarming

Some symptoms observed immediately after trauma are "normal" in the sense of affecting most survivors and being socially acceptable, psychologically effective, and self-limited. However, other symptoms may announce trouble. Among these are symptoms of dissociation, which—particularly when they repeat themselves after evacuation—should be seen as very alarming (Eriksson and Lundin 1996; Marmar et al. 1994; Shalev et al. 1996). Other symptoms may be predictive by their sheer intensity, yet studies have shown that the intensity of initial symptoms is not a specific predictor of PTSD (i.e., most people who express intense symptoms will still recover) (Shalev et al. 1997). The opposite, however, is very true: survivors who do not express a high degree of distress after traumatic events are more likely not to develop posttraumatic disorders. In other words, lack of significant distress has more predictive power than the presence of such symptoms.

Tolerance and Communicability of Symptoms

As mentioned above, a short period of shock and/or heroic defenses is regularly followed by repeated recollections of the traumatic event. Within this general pattern, some survivors are extremely disturbed, whereas others are not. The intrusive recollections, for example, may be so severe that they are fearfully avoided; are experienced as a torment; seriously interfere with sleep; curtail conversations about the traumatic event; create a wall of silence; and increase the survivor's isolation and loneliness. In other cases, however, survivors use the intrusive recollections to repeatedly tell others about the traumatic event and thereby recruit sympathy and help. Such repetitious retelling of the story is so frequent that it may be useful to educate primary caregivers, such as nurses and family members, to be tolerant to and accepting of hearing the same story again and again. A closer observation of the "effective" retelling of the story shows that its content changes with time—the narrative becomes richer, includes other elements, and takes a reflective tone (e.g., "when I think about it now, I could have done worse"). Nightmares are often changing as well, from mere repetition of one instance of the traumatic event to more remote renditions of the event associated with past events and with the person's total life experience. Such individuals may be on their way to recovery.

Specific Syndromes

Acute Stress Disorder

DSM-IV-TR (American Psychiatric Association 2000) proposes a diagnostic category of acute stress disorder (ASD) with symptoms of PTSD (reexperiencing, avoidance, and hyperarousal) occurring, along with dissociative symptoms, within 1 month of the traumatic event (Table 7–1). Although symptoms

---

TABLE 7-1.   DSM-IV-TR diagnostic criteria for acute stress disorder

---

A. The person has been exposed to a traumatic event in which both of the following were present:

   (1) the person experienced, witnessed, or was confronted with an event or events that involved actual or threatened death or serious injury, or a threat to the physical integrity of self or others

   (2) the person's response involved intense fear, helplessness, or horror

B. Either while experiencing or after experiencing the distressing event, the individual has three (or more) of the following dissociative symptoms:

   (1) a subjective sense of numbing, detachment, or absence of emotional responsiveness

   (2) a reduction in awareness of his or her surroundings (e.g., "being in a daze")

   (3) derealization

   (4) depersonalization

   (5) dissociative amnesia (i.e., inability to recall an important aspect of the trauma)

C. The traumatic event is persistently reexperienced in at least one of the following ways: recurrent images, thoughts, dreams, illusions, flashback episodes, or a sense of reliving the experience; or distress on exposure to reminders of the traumatic event.

D. Marked avoidance of stimuli that arouse recollections of the trauma (e.g., thoughts, feelings, conversations, activities, places, people).

E. Marked symptoms of anxiety or increased arousal (e.g., difficulty sleeping, irritability, poor concentration, hypervigilance, exaggerated startle response, motor restlessness).

F. The disturbance causes clinically significant distress or impairment in social, occupational, or other important areas of functioning or impairs the individual's ability to pursue some necessary task, such as obtaining necessary assistance or mobilizing personal resources by telling family members about the traumatic experience.

G. The disturbance lasts for a minimum of 2 days and a maximum of 4 weeks and occurs within 4 weeks of the traumatic event.

H. The disturbance is not due to the direct physiological effects of a substance (e.g., a drug of abuse, a medication) or a general medical condition, is not better accounted for by Brief Psychotic Disorder, and is not merely an exacerbation of a preexisting Axis I or Axis II disorder.

Source.   Reprinted from American Psychiatric Association: *Diagnostic and Statistical Manual of Mental Disorders*, 4th Edition, Text Revision. Washington, DC, American Psychiatric Association, 2000. Copyright 2000 American Psychiatric Association. Used with permission.

of ASD may occur at any time (including during the traumatic event), for the diagnosis to be made they should last for at least 2 days and should cause clinically significant distress, significantly interfere with the individual's functioning, or impair the individual's ability to pursue necessary tasks.

The presence of full or partial ASD may be associated with an increased risk of developing PTSD (Bryant and Harvey 1998; Classen et al. 1998; North et al. 1994). ASD has been linked with prior mental disorders (Barton et al. 1996). However, many survivors without initial ASD develop PTSD as well. Specifically, a subset of ASD symptoms (numbing, depersonalization, a sense of reliving the trauma, and motor restlessness) has been found to be strongly predictive of PTSD, whereas other symptoms, including most dissociative symptoms, did not (Harvey and Bryant 1998). Although the presence of ASD clearly signals a higher risk of developing PTSD, the validity of the currently defined syndrome has been questioned.

Dissociation and Depression

Symptoms of depression and dissociation have been evident in recent trauma survivors. Among injured survivors, dissociation during the traumatic event (peritraumatic dissociation) was found to be significantly associated with the subsequent development of PTSD (Shalev et al. 1996). Holen (1993) found that dissociation during the North Sea oil rig disaster was significantly associated with the short-term psychological outcome of survivors of this event. Bremner et al. (1992) found that Vietnam veterans with PTSD had experienced levels of dissociative symptoms during combat that were higher than those reported by veterans without PTSD. Koopman et al. (1994) found that early dissociative symptoms in survivors of the Oakland/Berkeley firestorm predicted PTSD symptoms 7 months later. Finally, Marmar et al. (1994) showed that peritraumatic dissociation in Vietnam veterans contributed to current PTSD over and above the contribution of combat exposure. Special emphasis should be given, therefore, to evaluating dissociative symptoms in survivors of any traumatic event.

Depression is often associated with chronic PTSD (Kessler et al. 1995) and might be an independent consequence of traumatic stress. Recent studies have shown that major depression occurs as early as 1 month after traumatization and that depressive symptoms 1 week after trauma and 1 month later predict chronic PTSD above and beyond the prediction made from PTSD and dissociation symptoms (Freedman et al. 1999). Although these data suggest that persistent depression in the weeks that follow trauma may require specific treatment intervention, not enough is known about the short-term and long-term effects of treating depression as such in the immediate aftermath of traumatic events.

Assessment and Evaluation

Given the problematic nature of assessing early symptoms, this chapter offers two alternatives: First, assessing the evolution of symptoms, and second, assessing the degree to which symptoms are tolerated by the survivor and the degree to which they interfere with normal functions or tasks. Beyond assessing symptoms, it is necessary to go back and evaluate risk factors related to the traumatic event; loss and damage incurred; presence of secondary stressors; quality, intensity, and development of the early responses; and availability of healing resources. A short overview of each of these domains follows.

The Traumatic Event

The assessment of the traumatic event should reveal what happened, what made an impact on the survivor. This information is easily obtained: trauma survivors tend to narrate their experience, often repeatedly, provided that confidence and safety have been established. The survivor's story, however, may be incomplete, mixed up, or redundant. One should listen to it and appraise its content and structure without confronting the subject with inconsistencies or interpretations. The story told includes concrete description, subjective appraisal, and emotional responses. As such it optimally represents the psychological reality of the event and the survivor's experience. Keeping a record of the initial narrative has tremendous value as testimony and for later ascertainment of facts and deeds.

Telling the story can be stressful, and it is rarely done without strong emotion. Telling the detail of the story to a helper is also binding, in that it creates an emotional bond between the narrator and the listener. Importantly, telling the story is an interaction, and good listeners are often those who respond emotionally while listening. Being in an interaction with survivors can be overwhelming for helpers, and it requires peer support and opportunity to ventilate and share emotions.

Loss and Damage Suffered

Traumatic events are often associated with real and symbolic losses. Among the former are loss of life, injury, loss of property, relocation, and loss of social network. Symbolic losses include loss of previously held beliefs and cognitive schemata and loss of one's identity, honor, and peace of mind. These have been authoritatively described elsewhere (Foa et al. 1989; Janoff-Bulman 1989; McCann and Pearlman 1992). Traumatized survivors often describe a loss of continuity with their previous life, such as "not being the same person anymore."

Facing losses may be the most distressing element of the immediate postimpact period of traumatic events. Importantly, recovery from loss involves grieving and readaptation, that is, new learning about self and others. Pharmacologic agents that interfere with learning (e.g., benzodiazepines) may prevent such learning. This explains preliminary data on the negative effect of administering such drugs continuously to trauma survivors (Gelpin et al. 1996)

Secondary Stressors

Traumatic events do not have a clear end point. Pain, uncertainty, and a series of surgical procedures may follow traumatic injury. This is especially true with burn victims (Taal and Faber 1997). Rape may be followed by aggressive police interrogation. Disasters are often the prelude of prolonged relocation, separation, and estrangement. Some survivors therefore are in the midst of continuous traumatization when helping efforts begin. These newly emerging adversities are referred to as secondary stressors.

Physiologic stressors may often go undetected in a recent survivor. Classic pitfalls include internal bleeding (e.g., in badly beaten rape victim) being mistaken for panic anxiety. Dehydration may be explained as mental confusion, or, conversely, agitation may be taken to be chemical intoxication (Ohbu et al. 1993). Pain is a major secondary stressor that has been linked with PTSD (Schreiber and Galai-Gat 1993). Medical examination must therefore precede the psychological assessment when the physical conditions of the trauma could have caused physical damage.

Countless psychological stressors may follow trauma. These can include bewilderment and disorientation, uncertainty about self and significant others, missing family members, or exposure to disfigured bodies or to other people's agony during evacuation. Helpers may systematize the quest for such stressors by asking the following simple questions: Is the survivor secure and out of danger? Does he or she have enough control over what is happening now? Are there major uncertainties in or around the patient's condition? Are negative events (or news) still expected? Does the patient have clear enough information about self and significant others? Has adequate human attention and warmth been given to the patient? Has trust been established between the patient and helpers? Can the current conditions humiliate or dishonor the patient?

Coping Efficacy

The assessment of coping efficacy takes the inquiry from the purely medical arena to the more general way of evaluating human performance and emotion. It will often be found that such a line of inquiry provides clinically relevant information. Four dimensions of successful coping are outlined above. Failure to cope, accordingly, may result in one or more of the following: impaired task performance (e.g., work, care of children, getting help), poorly modulated emotions (e.g., fear, sadness, anger), negative self-perception (e.g., self-accusation, self-devaluation), and the inability to enjoy rewarding interaction with others (including inability to be helped).

The clinician may wish to assess coping behavior during the traumatic event or current coping efficacy. The following questions may be of help in the assessment of global coping efficacy: Can the survivor continue task-oriented activity? How well organized, goal directed, and effective is such activity? Is the survivor overwhelmed by strong emotions most of the time? Can emotions be modulated when such modulation is required? Is the survivor inappropriately blaming himself or herself? Does the survivor generalize such accusations to his or her personality or self? How isolated, alienated, or withdrawn is the survivor? Does he or she seek the company of others or rather avoid it?

Interventions

Few individuals can pull themselves out of traumatic occurrences by their own will and power. The general case is that trauma survivors need help and support from others, and sometimes from those professionally trained to help. The latter often refer to their way of helping others as being a "treatment." To be effective, however, such treatment interventions must first meet the survivor's needs. Those who provide treatment must be tolerant of symptomatic behavior and respect the person's ability to self-regulate and monitor his or her environment. Importantly, the survivor must be able to properly utilize and enjoy what is offered. Stress responses may reduce such capacity, yet social or cultural mismatch between helpers and survivors may also reduce the usefulness of "treatment." Interventions should therefore be tuned to needs, capacities, and desires of survivors.

Generic Goals of Early Interventions

The first of the main goals of early intervention is to reduce psychobiological distress, which seems to be strongly related to subsequent psychopathology. Within this goal, reducing the effect of secondary stressors is often the precondition for conducting other interventions. Second, specific symptoms must be treated when they interfere with normal healing processes, that is, sharing and assimilating the traumatic event. And third, because situations of extreme stress are followed by natural healing processes, the best that therapy can do is to assist the normal healing, by supporting the survivor and his or her immediate helpers and by seeing that such helpers are available (e.g., making sure that families are evacuated together). In terms of assessment and evaluation, the main goal at this stage is to follow progress. Assessment of global coping efficacy functions may be a useful tool to follow such progress.

Interventions in the Different Phases
of the Acute Response

Peritraumatic Period

During this stage, the goal of interventions is to protect the survivors from further exposure to stress, contain the immediate physiologic and psychological responses, and increase controllability of the event and of subsequent rescue efforts.

Mental health professionals do not conduct most interventions at this stage. Yet some psychological principles apply. First, it is essential to maintain human contact with survivors throughout rescue efforts. Within human contacts, one should remember that survivors may have difficulty verbalizing their experiences; however, other bodily and emotional channels may be open for communication. Helpers should be tuned and responsive to the survivor's attempts to gain a degree of comfort and dignity during the event (e.g., by covering his or her body, avoiding intrusive looks of others and of the media).

Second, one should not spare efforts to soothe and comfort a recent survivor. Soothing bodily contacts with the recently rescued are often of great help, yet gender and social boundaries must be respected. Bringing in natural helpers (e.g., relatives) and helping them by advice and orientation may be of great help.

To increase controllability and reduce the unexpected, one should reorient the survivor within the rescuing environment. Rescuers should clearly identify themselves and their role. They should continuously inform the survivors about steps to be taken (e.g., evacuation to a hospital), medication to be given (e.g., morphine), and any other information. Although genuine information (including admitting a lack of information) must be the rule, breaking bad news may not be the rescuer's primary goal. A link between survivors from the same family should be established and, if possible, survivors should be evacuated along with those to whom they are close.

Finally, at this phase, those who participate in rescue efforts are also at risk for developing stress responses. Excessive self-exposure (e.g., being unable to disengage from work), irritability, inability to relax, and difficulties communicating with others are warning signs of burnout. A perception of having failed (e.g., by not preventing death or injury) is particularly poignant. Monitoring rescuers' exposure, securing and ordering resting periods, relieving overburdened workers, and conducting debriefings may help reduce the effect of traumatic stressors on rescuers.

Immediate Early Responses

Shortly after exposure, the traumatic event ceases to be a concrete event and starts to become a psychological event. As such, it has to be metabolized and assimilated, that is, it must become part of the survivor's inner network of meanings and experiences. Assimilating a traumatic event is often very painful and involves repeated recall and reassessment of the traumatic event and progressive assimilation. Progressive sensitization may also occur, in which aversive responses increase and are generalized to other psychological and social domains. The task of early intervention is therefore to facilitate psychological recovery and disable progressive sensitization.

Several mediators of recovery are well known at this point. These include verbalizing and sharing the individual story with others, being able to endure and express painful emotions, and oscillating between periods of extreme anguish and relative rest. Continuous distress, turning one's back to others, and being unable to think about the trauma (but rather experience it) are symptoms of bad processing.

A professional therapist is not needed when proper processing of the traumatic event takes place. Therefore, the first role of a therapist is to assess the strengths and the weaknesses of the survivor's immediate supporters.

One should allow for specific recovery styles to develop in individuals and families (one may talk and another may be silent). In some cases it is important to educate and explain the saliency of symptoms to survivors and their helpers. It is important to monitor the success or failure of a recovery style.

Emergence of Specific Symptoms

An interesting observation shows that burn victims as well as other injured trauma survivors (Baur et al. 1998; Shalev et al. 1993) become more symptomatic as they prepare to leave the hospital. Fully expressed phobic responses, major depression, and acute PTSD may indeed characterize the period of reentry to life, possibly because they start to interfere with normal tasks. At this time dedicated interventions are called for, including specific therapies (see below) and pharmacotherapy. One should be aware, however, that recovery is still the most frequent outcome, and that one is not yet treating a chronic posttraumatic stress disorder.

Specific Techniques

Despite the rich history of attempts to treat the immediate survivor, evidence regarding the long-term effect of early intervention is missing. The following are descriptions of methods used in the past to treat the immediate response to traumatization. Lack of empirical data in this area should not be confounded with negative results. The field is lacking prospective evaluations of trauma survivors, which could surely identify the best course of action.

Crisis Interventions and Stress Management

Stress theory suggests that the more distressed an individual is, the less capable he or she is to mentally disengage from the situation, reflect, imagine, and create solutions. Moreover, there is a natural tendency to repeat ineffectual attempts to solve a problem without changing them. Crisis interventions attempt to stop the vicious cycle of catastrophic appraisal and extreme distress. They also address the perception, by those in crisis, that their reaction is abnormal or that they have totally lost their inner strength.

In the recent survivor, crisis interventions address the elements of the short-term response to trauma that may not work effectively because of excessive distress. The situation of crisis is perceived as one in which the individual is caught in an emotional and cognitive trap, hence a "crisis." Crisis situations are emotionally overwhelming and cognitively inescapable. The survivor, accordingly, does not engage in effective salutary efforts and cannot perceive a solution to the situation, often despite adequate resources.

The combination of extreme distress and blindness to solutions is intolerable to most individuals and may result in unexpected behavior (e.g., suicide, life-threatening bravery). Statements such as "all is lost," "there is no way out," and "I can't tolerate it for another minute" are typical expressions of crises.

Crisis intervention starts by appraising with the individual (or the group) what, in a given situation, creates intolerable distress. It is often found that one specific element of the whole situation (e.g., lost communication with a family member) is most distressful. The second step is to recognize and legitimize, yet smoothly challenge, the perceived totality of the situation. Once this is clarified, one may address efforts already made to solve the salient problem and assess other ways or other resources. It is often found that once extreme emotions subside, individuals may find better solutions than expected. Solutions may include alternative plans of action, effective help-seeking, or postponing efforts to find a solution and engaging in alternative goals (e.g., "meanwhile I also have to take care of my children"). Moving subjects from a stage of disarray to a stage of effective coping signals the success of crisis intervention.

Treatment of Combat Stress Reaction Within the Military

Combat stress reaction (CSR) and its treatment have been authoritatively discussed elsewhere (e.g., Z. Solomon 1993). It is important to note that the goals assigned to the treatment of combat soldiers have never been purely medical and often included other considerations, such as reducing manpower loss due to psychological reactions. Within this dual goal, a strategy of frontline treatment has often been used. Otherwise known as the PIE model (for proximity, immediacy, and expectations), this treatment approach insisted on treating CSR casualties as soon as possible, as near as possible to the front line, and with an expectation of recovery and return to duty. The content of PIE interventions varied, going from a minimalist approach (known as the "chicken soup" treatment) in which protection, shelter, and respite were the main elements, to more active supportive group therapies.

Several controversial elements of the PIE model may still be in the back of one's mind when it comes to treating the acutely traumatized. First, one may be tempted to assume that in itself, an early return to "duty" or full performance is salutary. Accordingly, a traumatized police officer may be immediately sent to another stressful task as part of his or her "therapy." It is important to emphasize that the effectiveness of such practice has not been confirmed by studies of CSR. Quite to the contrary, the extensive "return to duty" policy, employed by United States psychiatrists in Vietnam (e.g., Bourne 1978), does not seem to have prevented the occurrence of PTSD. The Israeli experience, in contrast, seems to show that the implementation of the PIE model was a success (Z. Solomon et al. 1986). It is important to remember, however, that all Israeli wars were short (e.g., 3 weeks of fighting during the 1982 Lebanon war). Those who returned to their units, therefore, did not have to face heavy combat.

Another problematic concept is the so-called labeling theory, according to which making a diagnosis or otherwise telling survivors that they have a problem (e.g., by sending them back to a treatment facility) may be pathogenic. Ignoring an existing problem, however, may not be better. Clinicians must find a balanced path between refusal to recognize that one is ill and overdramatizing one's malady. Indeed, what seems to work in the frontline treatment is a natural selection process whereby those who recover within the time allocated to staying in a frontline facility may go back to their previous role, whereas those with persistent reactions are evacuated to the rear. In general, therefore, it may be wise to support the survivor in the immediate aftermath of traumatization and follow his or her progress before making a final assessment of severity.

Brief Cognitive Interventions

Cognitive-behavioral therapy (CBT) is an effective treatment for prolonged PTSD (see Chapter 3, in this volume). In the more recently traumatized, CBT has been evaluated in two controlled trials: Foa et al. (1995) evaluated a brief prevention program comprising four sessions for female victims of sexual and nonsexual assault. The intervention group was matched with a group of victims seen previously. At 2-month follow-up, the intervention group had a 10% rate of PTSD compared with 70% in the control group. Bryant et al. (1998) compared five sessions of CBT with sessions of supportive counseling in ASD. Seventeen percent of CBT patients and 67% of supportive counseling patients had PTSD at 6 months. Echeburua et al. (1996) similarly showed that cognitive restructuring and specific coping skills training was superior to relaxation training in reducing PTSD symptoms (but not other symptoms) at 12 months.

CBT-derived interventions, therefore, seem to be useful for acute stress disorder, that is, at the stage of early syndrome formation. However, the current literature provides no comparison between CBT and other active approaches (e.g., pharmacotherapy, intensive interpersonal psychotherapy). Thus, it would be inappropriate at this stage to say that only CBT works.

Debriefing

Debriefing has been developed as a semistructured group intervention designed to alleviate initial distress and prevent the development of mental disorders after exposure to traumatic events (Dyregrov 1989; Mitchell 1983; Raphael 1986). Debriefing usually consists of one session, during which the participants in an event share and learn from their experiences.

Among debriefing protocols, Mitchell's Critical Incident Stress Debriefing (CISD; Mitchell 1983), and a more recent version, Dyregrov's (1989) Psychological Debriefing, have been largely implemented. CISD sessions include seven consecutive stages: 1) introduction, in which the purpose of the session and its rules are described; 2) a fact phase, which consists of describing the traumatic event; 3) a thought phase addresses the appraisal of the event; 4) a reaction phase explores the participants' emotion during and after the event; 5) a symptom phase discusses the normal nature of symptoms; 6) a teaching phase prepares for future developments and outlines ways of coping with further consequences of the traumatic events; and 7) a reentry or disengagement phase offers a general discussion of the session and practical conclusions. The length of the sessions may vary. The same series of consecutive steps has been used in individual cases as well.

Debriefing sessions were expected to accomplish a great deal. Among the goals are reviewing the facts, sharing emotions, validating individual experiences, learning coping skills, evaluating current symptoms, and preparing for future experiences. The long-term objective of debriefing, which is the prevention of stress disorders, is also very ambitious. As shown in Table 7–2, however, controlled follow-up studies have not shown that debriefing has such capacity (Bisson and Deahl 1994; Bisson et al. 1997; Deahl et al. 1994; Hobbs et al.1996; Lee et al. 1996). Notwithstanding, the same studies show that most survivors perceived debriefing sessions as beneficial and satisfying. Moreover, debriefing has been shown to significantly reduce concurrent distress and enhance group cohesion (Shalev et al. 1998a). It is therefore too early to conclude that debriefing is of no use, mostly because no study has evaluated debriefing in a context of continuous care. What one may conclude, however, is that single-session interventions are not enough to stop the development of stress disorders.

Pharmacologic Interventions

Very little is known about the pharmacotherapy of recent trauma survivors. As with other forms of therapy, pharmacotherapy has two distinct targets: control of current distress and prevention of subsequent stress disorders. The two targets are often complementary, but they may also be contradictory (see discussion of benzodiazepines, below).

Current empirical research assigns two specific targets for early pharmacologic treatment: hyperarousal (including sleep disturbances) and depression. As discussed above, hyperarousal in the days and weeks after trauma predicts subsequent PTSD. Depressive symptoms 1 week after trauma were also found to predict PTSD at 4 months and at 1 year (Freedman et al. 1999). The role of anxiolytics and antidepressants is therefore discussed first.

Anxiolytics (mostly benzodiazepines) can reduce anxiety and improve sleep in recent trauma survivors. Their use, however, should be monitored: a study of prolonged treatment by high-potency benzodiazepines in recent trauma survivors (2–18 days after trauma) has shown that these drugs were associated with a higher incidence of PTSD at 6 months (Gelpin et al. 1996). On the other hand, Mellman et al. (1998) administered a benzodiazepine hypnotic for 5 nights to recent (between 1 and 3 weeks) trauma survivors and found an improvement in sleep and PTSD symptoms. The use of sedatives, therefore, should have a specific target (e.g., sleep, control of panic attacks) and should be time limited.

As shown in recent studies, chronic PTSD symptoms may be reduced by antidepressants (see Chapter 4, in this volume). Moreover, the effect of antidepressants may be greater in individuals with recent PTSD (van der

TABLE 7–2. Studies on the impact of debriefing

Study	Type of trauma (N)[a]	Time after trauma	Method	Outcome measures	Results
Bisson et al. 1997	Burn trauma (46/57)	2–19 days	Individual "debriefing" vs. no intervention	IES, HADS, CAPS	Negative effect at 13 months. Satisfaction in 52% of survivors
Hobbs et al. 1996	MVA victims (52/54)	<2 days	Individual "debriefing" vs. standard care	IES, BSI at 4 months	Worse outcome after interventions
Lee et al. 1996	Miscarriage (21/19)	2 weeks	Individual "debriefing" vs. no intervention	IES and HADS at 4 months	No significant effect by psychometrics. "Helpful" by clients' judgment
Deahl et al. 1994	Body handlers (20/40)	Misc.	Group debriefing	IES, GHQ-28 at 9 months	No effect
Rose et al. 1999	Assault victims		PD/psychoeducation/no treatment (54/52/51)	PSS, IES, BDI	No difference at all between groups at 11 months
Deahl et al. 2000	Peacekeeping force in Bosnia/assessments control subjects (54/52)		Group debriefing	IES, HADS	Lower anxiety in PD group; greater reduction in PTSD symptoms among control subjects
Mayou et al. 2000	Motor vehicle accident survivors		Follow-up of Hobbs et al. 1996 at 3 years	BSI, IES, travel anxiety, financial status, overall functioning	PD group has worse outcome across measures. No difference in PTSD symptoms

Note. BDI=Beck Depression Inventory; BSI=Brief Symptom Inventory; CAPS=Clinician-Administered PTSD Scale; GHQ-28=General Health Questionnaire; HADS=Hamilton Depression Scale; IES=Impact of Events Scale; MVA=motor vehicle accident; PSS=PTSD Symptom Scale.
[a]Numbers in parentheses are the number of subjects who received treatment and the number of control subjects.

Kolk et al. 1994). Given the above-mentioned association between early depression and PTSD (Freedman et al. 1999), it is not unreasonable to use antidepressants in the treatment of posttraumatic depression. Among antidepressants, one may prefer those that have been shown to affect chronic PTSD. It is important to follow up on patients and monitor the effect of antidepressants. Treatment may be started during the first weeks after trauma. When depression is not present, however, the rationale for using antidepressants is not very strong, yet these drugs have been shown to affect core PTSD symptoms in patients with prolonged disorders. Clearly, treatment with antidepressants should be reserved for the period in which specific syndromes are expressed and is not currently justified in the treatment of the immediate response.

Future and Hypothetical Approaches

Current theories of causation assign several additional and yet hypothetical targets. First, PTSD may result from neuronal kindling (Post et al. 1997), hence the hypothetical usefulness of antikindling drugs, such as valproate, in the early aftermath of traumatization. Second, PTSD has been associated with sympathetic activation during and immediately after trauma (Shalev et al. 1998b). Sympathetic activation has also been associated with increased recall of negative emotions. Hypothetically, therefore, drugs that reduce sympathetic activation, such as propranolol, have been proposed as immediate preventive treatment in recent trauma survivors. The administration of propranolol should start as soon as possible after trauma (i.e., on admission to an emergency room). Third, PTSD has been associated with a cascade of biological events related to the activation of corticotropin-release hormone (CRH) receptors in central brain nuclei. Modulators of CRH activity may become available and my be used in the future for the prevention of PTSD. Finally, chronic PTSD has been associated with cortisol-related damage to hippocampal cells. Several compounds were found to protect the hippocampus from cortisol-related cellular damage, and these drugs may be of use in PTSD as well.

Conclusion

Early interventions after trauma are not easy to conduct. Controlled prospective studies of such interventions are even more difficult and raise both practical and ethical problems. Consequently, the uncertainty about the long-term effects of early interventions is likely to remain. Lessons from the recent and not-so-recent past do not show that early interventions can prevent PTSD. Such is the case in the Vietnam and the Lebanon wars, where the management of combat stress responses was seen as an important service to combatants. Such is also the case in most studies of debriefing, as cited above.

There are multiple reasons for such unfortunate results, probably the first among which is the complex etiology of PTSD, which encompasses biological endowment, acquired vulnerability, intensity of traumatization, and recovery factors. Within such a complex etiology, the relative contribution of early and short interventions is necessarily small. Other reasons to believe that the task of preventing stress disorders is indeed tremendous are outlined in this chapter. These include the plasticity of the early reaction, the admixture of normal and abnormal behavior, the difficulties in identifying subjects at risk, and the proper difficulties of conducting interventions in the early aftermath of disastrous events.

Still, knowledge accumulated so far leads to reducing the above-mentioned uncertainties. First, convincing success of some interventions has been documented recently, mainly through the use of cognitive-behavioral techniques. This is an important step forward, which should be followed. Central to pursuing this venue is the question of timing of the intervention. Studies of CBT have been conducted in the weeks after traumatic events, and not during the first few days. Possibly other treatment methods may be useful at later stages, such as treatment for depression, which has been shown to strongly predict PTSD.

If effective treatment can be administered during the early posttraumatic period, then it is mandatory to deliver it to symptomatic survivors. What the immediate contact can provide the survivor is an open door (or address) for continuous treatment and the ability to identify oneself as being in need of treatment. Short contacts during the immediate aftermath of traumatization therefore should end by advising survivors about possible sources of help and about self-diagnosis. In addition, survivors should be systematically evaluated at the end of treatment so that those who are abnormally symptomatic will have knowledge of their situation and receive additional treatment. What constitute abnormal symptoms is obviously a matter of clinical judgment. The coping model proposed above, or indeed any measure of the interference of symptoms with expected performance may facilitate such judgment.

As to the earlier stages of the immediate response to traumatic events, the following sequence suggests a general framework. At first provide concrete help, food, warmth, and shelter. Once the survivor is out of concrete danger, immediate treatment is mainly by soothing and reducing states of extreme emotion and increasing controllability. At a third stage, survivors have to be assisted in the painful and repetitive reappraisal of the trauma. The appropriate level of clinical observation and decision making at this stage may be the salient symptom (e.g., pain, insomnia). Treating specific syndromes comes at the following stage, when syndromes can be reliably diagnosed and observed. Acute PTSD, depression, and possibly other anxiety disorders are the main targets for treatment at this stage.

Finally, one should look forward to further discovery in the area of early responses and their treatment. Studies of chemical agents (e.g., propranolol) are now on their way. Attention given to traumatization may lead to trials of additional immediate therapies. Better understanding of predictors and risk factors for chronic disorders may enable more valid diagnostic routines in the future. Yet, preventing stress disorders is only one goal of early interventions. Providing immediate relief is not a lesser task. Possibly the two should not be confounded, and one should help those who suffer at the level of their immediate human and clinical needs while simultaneously hoping to prevent chronic stress disorders.

References

American Psychiatric Association: Diagnostic and Statistical Manual of Mental Disorders, 4th Edition. Washington, DC, American Psychiatric Association, 1994

American Psychiatric Association: Diagnostic and Statistical Manual of Mental Disorders, 4th Edition, Text Revision. Washington, DC, American Psychiatric Association, 2000

Antelman SM: Time-dependent sensitization as the cornerstone for a new approach to pharmacotherapy: drugs as foreign/stressful stimuli. Drug Development Research 14:1–30, 1988

Barton KA, Blanchard EB, Hickling EJ: Antecedents and consequences of acute stress disorder among motor vehicle accident victims. Behav Res Ther 34:805–813, 1996

Baur KM, Hardy PE, Van Dorsten B: Posttraumatic stress disorder in burn populations: a critical review of the literature. J Burn Care Rehabil 19:230–240, 1998

Bisson JI, Deahl MP: Psychological debriefing and prevention of post-traumatic stress—more research is needed. Br J Psychiatry 165:717–720, 1994

Bisson JI, Jenkins PL, Alexander J, et al: Randomised controlled trial of psychological debriefing for victims of acute burn trauma. Br J Psychiatry 171:78–81, 1997

Blanchard EB, Hickling EJ, Forneris CA, et al: Prediction of remission of acute posttraumatic stress disorder in motor vehicle accident victims. J Trauma Stress 10:215–234, 1997

Bland SH, O'Leary ES, Farinaro E, et al: Social network disturbances and psychological distress following earthquake evacuation. J Nerv Ment Dis 185:188–194, 1997

Bourne PG: Military psychiatry and the Viet Nam War in perspective, in The Psychology and Physiology of Stress. Edited by Bourne PG. New York, Academic Press, 1978, pp 219–236

Bremner JD, Southwick S, Brett E, et al: Dissociation and posttraumatic stress disorder in Vietnam combat veterans. Am J Psychiatry 149:328–332, 1992

Breslau N, Davis GC: Posttraumatic stress disorder in an urban population of young adults: risk factors for chronicity. Am J Psychiatry 149:671–675, 1992

Bryant RA, Harvey AG: Relationship between acute stress disorder and posttraumatic stress disorder following mild traumatic brain injury. Am J Psychiatry 155:625–629, 1998

Bryant RA, Harvey AG, Dang ST, et al: Treatment of acute stress disorder: a comparison of cognitive-behavioral therapy and supportive counseling. J Consult Clin Psychol 66(5):862–866, 1998

Cahill L, Prins B, Weber M, et al: Beta-adrenergic activation and memory for emotional events. Nature 371:702–704, 1994

Classen C, Koopman C, Hales R, et al: Acute stress disorder as a predictor of posttraumatic stress symptoms. Am J Psychiatry 155:620–624, 1998

Dasberg H: Belonging and loneliness in relation to mental breakdown in battle. Israel Annals of Psychiatry and Related Disciplines 14:307–321, 1976

Deahl MP, Gillham AB, Thomas J, et al: Psychological sequelae following the Gulf War. Factors associated with subsequent morbidity and the effectiveness of psychological debriefing. Br J Psychiatry 165:60–65, 1994

Deahl M, Srinivasan M, Jones N, et al: Preventing psychological trauma in soldiers: the role of operational stress training and psychological debriefing. Br J Med Psychol 73:77–85, 2000

Dyregrov A: Caring for helpers in disaster situations: psychological debriefing. Disaster Management 2:25–30, 1989

Echeburua E, De Corral P, Sarasua B, et al: Treatment of acute posttraumatic stress disorder in rape victims: an experimental study. J Anxiety Disord 10:185–199, 1996

Ehlers A, Clark DM, Dunmore E, et al: Predicting response to exposure treatment in PTSD: the role of mental defeat and alienation. J Trauma Stress 11:457–471, 1998a

Ehlers A, Mayou RA, Bryant B: Psychological predictors of chronic posttraumatic stress disorder after motor vehicle accidents. J Abnorm Psychol 107:508–519, 1998b

Eriksson NG, Lundin T: Early traumatic stress reactions among Swedish survivors of the m/s Estonia disaster. Br J Psychiatry 169:713–716, 1996

Foa EB, Steketee G, Rothbaum BO: Behavioral/cognitive conceptualizations of post-traumatic stress disorder. Behavior Therapy 20:155–176, 1989

Foa EB, Zinbarg R, Rothbaum BO: Uncontrollability and unpredictability in post-traumatic stress disorder: an animal model. Psychol Bull 112:218–238, 1992

Foa EB, Hearst-Ikeda D, Perry KJ: Evaluation of a brief cognitive-behavioral program for the prevention of chronic PTSD in recent assault victims. J Consult Clin Psychol 63:948–955, 1995

Freedman SA, Brandes D, Peri T, et al: Predictors of chronic PTSD—a prospective study. Br J Psychiatry 174:353–359, 1999

Freud S: Beyond the pleasure principles (1920), in The Standard Edition of the Complete Works of Sigmund Freud, Vol 18. Translated and edited by Strachey J. London, Hogarth Press, 1957, p 64

Gelpin E, Bonne O, Peri T, et al: Treatment of recent trauma survivors with benzodiazepines: a prospective study. J Clin Psychiatry 57:390–394, 1996

Green BL: Defining trauma: terminology and generic stressors dimensions. Journal of Applied Social Psychology 20:1632–1642, 1995

Harvey AG, Bryant RA: The relationship between acute stress disorder and posttraumatic stress disorder: a prospective evaluation of motor vehicle accident survivors. J Consult Clin Psychol 66:507–512, 1998

Hobbs M, Mayou R, Harrison B, et al: A randomised controlled trial of psychological debriefing for victims of road traffic accidents. BMJ 313:1438–1439, 1996

Hobfoll SE, Jackson AP: Conservation of resources in community intervention. Am J Community Psychol 19:111–121, 1991

Holen A: The North Sea oil rig disaster, in International Handbook of Traumatic Stress Syndromes. Edited by Wilson JP, Raphael B. New York, Plenum, 1993, pp 471–478

Janoff-Bulman R: Shattered Assumption: Towards a New Psychology of Trauma. New York, Free Press, 1992

Kessler RC, Sonnega A, Bromet E, et al: Posttraumatic stress disorder in the National Comorbidity Survey. Arch Gen Psychiatry 52:1048–1060, 1995

Koopman C, Classen C, Spiegel D: Predictors of posttraumatic stress symptoms among survivors of the Oakland/Berkeley, Calif, firestorm. Am J Psychiatry 151:888–894, 1994

Kormos HR: The Nature of Combat Stress in Combat Stress Disorders Among Vietnam Veterans. Edited by Figley C. New York, Brunner/Mazel, 1978, pp 3–22

Kozaric Kovacic D, Folnegovic Smalc V, Marusic A: Acute post-traumatic stress disorder in prisoners of war released from detention camps. Drustvena Istrazivanja 7:485–497, 1998

Lazarus RS, Folkman S: Cognitive appraisal processes, in Stress, Appraisal and Coping. New York, Springer, 1984, pp 22–54

Lee C, Slade P, Lygo V: The influence of psychological debriefing on emotional adaption in women following early miscarriage: a preliminary study. Br J Med Psychol 69:47–58, 1996

Lindemann E: Symptomatology and management of acute grief: 1944. Am J Psychiatry 151:155–160, 1994

Loftus EF: The reality of repressed memories. Am Psychol 48:518–537, 1993

Marmar CR, Weiss DS, Schlenger WE, et al: Peritraumatic dissociation and posttraumatic stress in male Vietnam theater veterans. Am J Psychiatry 151:902–907, 1994

Mayou R, Ehlers A, Hobbs M: Psychological debriefing for road traffic accident victims: three-year follow-up of a randomized controlled trial. Br J Psychiatry 176:589–593, 2000

McCann IL, Pearlman LA: Constructivist self-development theory: a theoretical framework for assessing and treating traumatized college students. J Am Coll Health 40:189–196, 1992

McCarroll JE, Ursano RJ, Fullerton CS: Symptoms of PTSD following recovery of war dead: 13–15-month follow-up. Am J Psychiatry 152:939–941, 1995

McGaugh JL: Significance and remembrance: the role of neuromodulatory systems. Psychological Sciences 1:15–25, 1990

Mellman TA, Byers PM, Augenstein JS: Pilot evaluation of hypnotic medication during acute traumatic stress response. J Trauma Stress 11:563–569, 1998

Metcalfe J, Jacobs WJ: A "hot-system/cool-system" view of memory under stress. PTSD Research Quarterly 7:1–3, 1996

Mitchell JT: When disaster strikes.... Journal of Emergency Medical Services 8:36–39, 1983

Munch A, Guyere PM, Holbrook MJ: Physiological functions of glucocorticoids in stress and their relations to pharmacological actions. Endocr Rev 93:9783–9799, 1984

North CS, Smith EM, Spitznagel EL: Posttraumatic stress disorder in survivors of a mass shooting. Am J Psychiatry 151:82–88, 1994

Ohbu S, Yamashina A, Takasu N, et al: Sarin poisoning on Tokyo subway. South Med J 90:587–593, 1993

Pearlin LI, Schooler C: The structure of coping. J Health Soc Behav 19(1):2–21, 1978

Pitman RK: Post-traumatic stress disorder, conditioning, and network theory. Psychiatric Annals 18:182–189, 1988

Post RM, Weiss SR., Smith M, et al: Kindling versus quenching. Implications for the evolution and treatment of posttraumatic stress disorder. Ann N Y Acad Sci 821:285–295, 1997

Prince CR, Anisman H: Situation specific effects of stressor controllability on plasma corticosterone changes in mice. Pharmacol Biochem Behav 37:613–621, 1990

Raphael B: When Disaster Strikes. New York, Basic Books, 1986, pp 222–244

Raphael B, Meldrum L, McFarlane AC: Does debriefing after psychological trauma work? time for randomised controlled trials. Accident and Emergency Nursing 4:65–67, 1996

Resnick HS, Yehuda R., Pitman RK, et al: Effect of previous trauma on acute plasma cortisol level following rape. Am J Psychiatry 152:1675–1677, 1995

Rose S, Brewin CR, Andrews B, et al: A randomized controlled trial of individual psychological debriefing for victims of violent crime. Psychol Med 29:793–799, 1999

Rosser R, Dewar S: Therapeutic flexibility in the post disaster response (editorial). J R Soc Med 84:2–3, 1991

Rothbaum BO, Foa EB: Subtypes of posttraumatic stress disorder and duration of symptoms, in Posttraumatic Stress Disorder, DSM-IV and Beyond. Edited by Davidson JRT, Foa EB. Washington, DC, American Psychiatric Press, 1993, pp 23–35

Schreiber S, Galai-Gat T: Uncontrolled pain following physical injury as the core-trauma in post-traumatic stress disorder. Pain 54:107–110, 1993

Shalev AY: Psychophysiological risk-factors for PTSD, in Risk Factors for PTSD. Edited by Yehuda R. Washington, DC, American Psychiatric Press, 1999, pp 143–162

Shalev AY, Rogel Fuchs Y, Pitman RK: Conditioned fear and psychological trauma. Biol Psychiatry 31:863–865, 1992

Shalev AY, Schreiber S, Galai T: Early psychiatric responses to traumatic injury. J Trauma Stress 6:441–450, 1993

Shalev AY, Peri T, Canetti L, et al: Predictors of PTSD in injured trauma survivors: a prospective study. Am J Psychiatry 153:219–225, 1996

Shalev AY, Freedman S, Peri T, et al: Predicting PTSD in trauma survivors: prospective evaluation of self-report and clinician-administered instruments. Br J Psychiatry 170:558–564, 1997

Shalev AY, Peri T, Rogel Fuchs Y, et al: Historical group debriefing after combat exposure. Mil Med 163(7):494–498, 1998a

Shalev AY, Sahar T, Freedman S, et al: A prospective study of heart rate response following trauma and the subsequent development of posttraumatic stress disorder. Arch Gen Psychiatry 55:553–559, 1998b

Shalev AY, Pitman RK, Orr SP, et al: Auditory startle in trauma survivors with PTSD: a prospective study. Am J Psychiatry 157:255–261, 2000

Solomon SD, Gerrity ET, Muff AM, et al: Efficacy of treatments for posttraumatic stress disorder. JAMA 268(5):633–638, 1992

Solomon Z: Combat Stress Reaction. New York, Plenum, 1993

Solomon Z, Benbenishty R: The role of proximity, immediacy, and expectancy in frontline treatment of combat stress reaction among Israelis in the Lebanon War. Am J Psychiatry 143:613–617, 1986

Solomon Z, Mikulincer M, Avitzur E: Coping, locus of control, social support, and combat-related posttraumatic stress disorder: a prospective study. J Pers Soc Psychol 55:279–285, 1988

Taal LA, Faber AW: Burn injuries, pain and distress: exploring the role of stress symptomatology. Burns 23:288–290, 1997

van der Kolk BA, Dreyfuss D, Michaels M, et al: Fluoxetine in posttraumatic stress disorder. J Clin Psychiatry 55:517–522, 1994

Yehuda R, McFarlane AC: Conflict between current knowledge about posttraumatic stress disorder and its original conceptual basis. Am J Psychiatry 152:1705–1713, 1995

Yehuda R, Southwick SM, Nussbaum G, et al: Low urinary cortisol excretion in patients with posttraumatic stress disorder. J Nerv Ment Dis 178:366–369, 1990

Yehuda R, McFarlane AC, Shalev AY: Predicting the development of posttraumatic stress disorder from the acute response to a traumatic event. Biol Psychiatry 44:1305–1313, 1998

Yitzhaki T, Solomon Z, Kotler M: The clinical picture of acute combat stress reaction among Israeli soldiers in the 1982 Lebanon War. Mil Med 156:193–197, 1991

Index

*Page numbers in **boldface** type refer to tables or figures.*